Minimal Residual Disease Testing

Todd E. Druley
Editor

Minimal Residual Disease Testing

Current Innovations and Future Directions

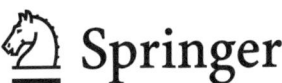

Editor
Todd E. Druley, MD, PhD
Department of Pediatrics
Washington University in St. Louis
St. Louis, MO
USA

ISBN 978-3-319-94826-3   ISBN 978-3-319-94827-0   (eBook)
https://doi.org/10.1007/978-3-319-94827-0

Library of Congress Control Number: 2018957568

© Springer International Publishing AG, part of Springer Nature 2019
This work is subject to copyright. All rights are reserved by the Publisher, whether the whole or part of the material is concerned, specifically the rights of translation, reprinting, reuse of illustrations, recitation, broadcasting, reproduction on microfilms or in any other physical way, and transmission or information storage and retrieval, electronic adaptation, computer software, or by similar or dissimilar methodology now known or hereafter developed.
The use of general descriptive names, registered names, trademarks, service marks, etc. in this publication does not imply, even in the absence of a specific statement, that such names are exempt from the relevant protective laws and regulations and therefore free for general use.
The publisher, the authors, and the editors are safe to assume that the advice and information in this book are believed to be true and accurate at the date of publication. Neither the publisher nor the authors or the editors give a warranty, express or implied, with respect to the material contained herein or for any errors or omissions that may have been made. The publisher remains neutral with regard to jurisdictional claims in published maps and institutional affiliations.

This Springer imprint is published by the registered company Springer Nature Switzerland AG
The registered company address is: Gewerbestrasse 11, 6330 Cham, Switzerland

Contents

1 **Introduction** 1
   Nitin Mahajan and Todd E. Druley

2 **Minimal Residual Disease Testing in Acute Lymphoblastic Leukemia/Lymphoma** 23
   Laura Wake, Xueyan Chen, and Michael J. Borowitz

3 **Molecular Diagnostics for Minimal Residual Disease Analysis in Hematopoietic Malignancies** ... 69
   Barbara K. Zehentner

4 **Monitoring AML Response Using "Difference from Normal" Flow Cytometry** 101
   Michael R. Loken, Lisa Eidenschink Brodersen, and Denise A. Wells

5 **ML-DS: A Unique Condition for Measurable Residual Disease Detection** 139
   Elisabeth R. Wilson and R. Spencer Tong

6 **Advancements in Next-Generation Sequencing for Detecting Minimal Residual Disease** 159
   Erin L. Crowgey and Nitin Mahajan

Index 193

Contributors

Michael J. Borowitz Department of Pathology, Johns Hopkins Medical Institutions, Baltimore, MD, USA

Lisa Eidenschink Brodersen Hematologics, Inc., Seattle, WA, USA

Xueyan Chen Department of Pathology, University of Washington, Seattle, WA, USA

Erin L. Crowgey Nemours Alfred I. duPont Hospital for Children, Biomedical Research Department, Wilmington, DE, USA

Todd E. Druley Washington University in St. Louis, Division of Hematology and Oncology, Department of Pediatrics, Center for Genome Sciences and Systems Biology, Saint Louis, MO, USA

Michael R. Loken Hematologics, Inc., Seattle, WA, USA

Nitin Mahajan Washington University in St. Louis, Pediatric Hematology and Oncology, St. Louis, MO, USA

R. Spencer Tong Washington University School of Medicine, Department of Pediatrics, St. Louis, ON, USA

Laura Wake Department of Pathology, Johns Hopkins Medical Institutions, Baltimore, MD, USA

Denise A. Wells Hematologics, Inc., Seattle, WA, USA

Elisabeth R. Wilson Hematologics Inc., Seattle, WA, USA

Washington University in St. Louis, Department of Biological and Biomedical Sciences, St. Louis, MO, USA

Barbara K. Zehentner Hematologics Inc., Seattle, WA, USA

Chapter 1
Introduction

Nitin Mahajan and Todd E. Druley

The detection of minimal residual disease (MRD) – or more aptly named measurable residual disease – has evolved substantially over recent decades with the steady improvement of technology. From gross morphology to karyotyping to cytogenetics to flow cytometry, MRD has matured and saved countless lives in the process by identifying those who require augmented therapy in order to overcome refractory or relapsed leukemia. New technologies, particularly with respect to DNA and RNA sequencing, offer such extreme sensitivity that focus has shifted to being certain that the mutation(s) detected is indeed representative of the leukemia population and not an incidental finding. Even healthy individuals harbor a rich profile of clonal hematopoietic

---

N. Mahajan
Washington University in St. Louis, Pediatric Hematology and Oncology, St. Louis, MO, USA

T. E. Druley (✉)
Washington University in St. Louis, Division of Hematology and Oncology, Department of Pediatrics, Center for Genome Sciences and Systems Biology, Saint Louis, MO, USA
e-mail: druley_t@wustl.edu

mutations [1] that is not fully understood and could lead to false positives without careful calibration. This is a concern for using cell-free or circulating tumor DNA in solid tumors as markers for metastatic or recurrent cancer.

This text is intended to not only review the history of methods utilized for MRD but also summarize the current state of the art as well as predict where MRD will move in the coming years. Clearly, with the rapid decline in sequencing costs coupled with the massive amounts of data generated, it will be sequencing strategies – both in bulk and in single cells – that dominate MRD in the near future. To that end, it seems appropriate to offer a brief history of nucleic acid sequencing and highlight some of the emerging sequencing platforms that are most likely to change the way laboratories and physicians order and view MRD.

History of DNA Sequencing

In year 1910, Albrecht Kossel discovered nucleotide bases adenine, cytosine, guanine, thymine, and uracil as the building block of nucleic acid [2]. Four decades later, Erwin Chargaff recognized the pairing pattern of these nucleotides in DNA and RNA [2]. Robert Holley and colleagues (1965) were accredited for sequencing the first ever full nucleic acid molecule, 77-nucleotide yeast (*Saccharomyces cerevisiae*) alanine tRNA with a proposed cloverleaf structure [3]. It took more than 5 years to extract enough tRNA from the yeast to identify the sequence of nucleotide residues using selective ribonuclease treatment, two-dimensional chromatography, and spectrophotometric procedures [3]. The laborious and expensive nature of the sequencing did not deter the scientists but rather drove the continuous development and refinement of sequencing methods. Initially, scientists focused sequencing efforts on the readily available populations of RNA species because (i) of bulk production in culture, (ii) it is not complicated by a complementary strand, and (iii) it is considerably thought to be shorter than DNA molecules [4, 5].

Fred Sanger and colleagues at Cambridge were one of the groups actively working on methods for sequencing DNA molecules. They developed a technique based on the detection of radiolabeled partial digestion fragments after two-dimensional fractionation [6], allowing addition of nucleotides to the growing pool of ribosomal and transfer RNA sequences. Using a primer extension method, Ray Wu and Dale Kaiser sequenced a short sequence of DNA for the first time [7]. However, the actual determination of bases was still restricted to small sequences of DNA because of the labor and use of radioactive and hazardous chemicals. These continuous efforts resulted in generating the first complete protein-coding gene sequence, coat protein of bacteriophage MS2 in 1972 [8], and the first complete 3569-nucleotide-long genome sequence of the bacteriophage MS2 RNA in 1976 [9].

Two influential techniques in the mid-1970s emerged which later gave a new dimension to the field of molecular biology. The two techniques were Alan Coulson and Sanger's "plus and minus" system and Allan Maxam and Walter Gilbert's chemical cleavage technique [10–12]. Both these techniques used polyacrylamide gel electrophoresis, which provided better resolving power, instead of previously used 2-D fractionation that often consisted of both electrophoresis and chromatography. The plus and minus technique was based on the addition of radiolabeled nucleotides next to the primer using DNA polymerase.

A "plus" reaction is where only a single type of nucleotide is present with an aim that all extensions will end with that particular nucleotide whereas a "minus" reaction three nucleotides are used to produce sequences up to the position before the next missing nucleotide. This led Sanger and colleagues to sequence the first DNA genome, that of bacteriophage [11]. On the other hand, the technique used by Maxam and Gilbert to sequence the DNA was quite different, as they used chemicals to fragment the radiolabeled DNA at particular bases. Fragmented radiolabeled DNA was electrophoresed through a polyacrylamide gel and based on the length of the cleaved fragments the sequence was inferred. Development of these two methods can be described as the foundation of modern sequencing. However, the major discovery in the field of DNA sequencing came in 1977 with the Sanger's "chain-termination" or "dideoxy technique," and since then it is the most widely used sequencing method.

The chain-termination technique utilizes labeled (radioactively or fluorescently) chemical analogues of the deoxynucleotides (dNTPs), which are called dideoxynucleotides (ddNTPs). The reaction includes a single-stranded DNA template, DNA primer, DNA polymerase, normal deoxynucleotides (dNTPs), and modified dideoxynucleotides (ddNTPs). Because ddNTPs lack a 3'-OH group, they are unable to make phosphodiester bond which ultimately terminates DNA strand elongation. A total of four DNA sequencing reactions are made, and in each reaction, three normal dNTPs and one labeled ddNTP are added. This results in the synthesis of each possible length of the DNA molecule of interest. The nucleotide sequence is inferred by resolving the product from each reaction in a separate lane of a polyacrylamide gel. Initially, scientists were able to determine the sequence of a molecule up to 300 bp.

The potential Sanger sequencing was realized quickly by the scientific community, and a series of improvements were made in the following years. Major improvements were, first, replacement of radioactive materials with fluorescent-based detection, which allowed the reaction to occur in one vessel instead of four. A second key improvement was the use of capillary-based electrophoresis which provided better resolution, required less equipment space, and decreased the amount of time required for the experiment. Following these improvements, Smith et al. (1986) at Applied Biosystems Instruments (ABI) designed an automated machinery to complete this procedure and later introduced the first commercial automated DNA sequencer [13].

First-generation sequencers incorporated a computer-based data acquisition and analysis and were capable of producing reads >300 bp. However, to analyze longer DNA molecules, "shotgun sequencing" was developed by separately cloning and sequencing overlapping DNA fragments. After sequencing these molecules are assembled into one long contiguous sequence [14]. The discovery of polymerase chain reaction (PCR) technology during this time period provided a viable solution for generating high concentrations of specific DNA species and aided in the re-sequencing of particular regions. With the addition of newer technologies and increased interest in sequencing, ABI sequencers were significantly improved over the next few years. These improvements included an increase in the number of lanes in gel-based models from 1 (ABI 310) to 16 (ABI 370A) and then to 96 (ABI 377). At the same time, the length of the reads increased from 350 (ABI 370A) to over 900 (ABI 3730xl), while the run times decreased from 18 h to 3 h [15].

The Institute for Genomic Research (TIGR) in Rockville, Maryland, founded by J. Craig Venter in 1992, pioneered the industrialization of an automated sequencer, with a focus on studying various genomes [16, 17]. With the establishment of both the first Affymetrix and GeneChip microarrays in 1996, expression studies involving various genes in prokaryotes and eukaryotes were now possible [18]. By the end of 1999, with continuous effort of various researchers, TIGR generated 83 million nucleotides of cDNA sequence, 87,000 human cDNA sequences, and the complete genome sequences of *Haemophilus influenzae* [19] and *Mycoplasma genitalium* [20].

With the beginning of the new century, though expensive and time-consuming, sequencing centers and international consortiums, such as the TIGR in the USA, the Sanger Centre in the UK, and RIKEN in Japan, using the automated sequencers, produced the complete sequence of the human genome. Additionally, the genomes of *Escherichia coli*, *Bacillus subtilis*, *Saccharomyces cerevisiae*, *Caenorhabditis elegans* (nematode), *Drosophila melanogaster* (fruit fly), and the plant *Arabidopsis thaliana* were also completed [4, 15, 17, 21]. Despite all these accomplishments, new sequencing methods continued to emerge with the aim to reduce costs, increase multiplexing, decrease time, and increase throughput.

Ultimately these improved methods have been realized over the past few decades and have paved the path forward for next-generation sequencing applications.

Next-Generation Sequencing Application

As advancements were being realized in sequencing applications, often referred to as next-generation sequencing (NGS), key improvements included (i) the parallelization of high number of sequencing reactions, (ii) the preparation of amplified sequencing libraries prior to sequencing, (iii) library amplification on miniature surfaces (solid surfaces, beads, emulsion droplets), (iv) direct monitoring of the nucleotides, (v) reduced cost, and (vi) decreased time.

There are a wide variety of NGS applications that can be used to study the whole genome, coding regions (exomes), transcriptome, DNA methylation, mitochondrial DNA, plus several other novel applications, such as micro-RNA and noncoding RNA sequencing. Sequencing applications for RNA are similar to that of DNA, with an additional step to generate cDNA from RNA using a reverse transcriptase. For targeted sequencing the exomes or regions of interest within the fragmented DNA can be captured and enriched by probe hybridization or by customized PCR amplification. Targeted panel sequencing involves a focused approach on known alleles of gene candidates, associated with the phenotype of interest.

The general workflow for an NGS assay involves (1) the isolation of nucleic acids (DNA or RNA), (2) the capture of DNA molecules of interest, (3) sequencing, and (4) bioinformatics analysis of the massive unstructured dataset [5, 17, 22, 23]. The exact procedures involved in each of these steps vary between sequencing platforms and library preparation protocols. Ultimately, since the genetics of cancer is extremely heterogeneous, it will be essential to use the appropriate technique for the type of variant of interest. Like instrumentation and protocols, the revision of read lengths occurs rapidly and will likely continue to do so as chemistries are optimized and improved. Determining an appropriate read length for sequencing, short versus long, depends on the goal of the experiment.

Long-read sequencing (LRS) techniques have been key for phasing studies and alternative splicing. However, as short-read sequencing (SRS) technologies advance in the single-cell sequencing field, these types of analysis will be more easily attended with SRS technology. Short-read sequencing (SRS) typically produces reads that are 50–600 bp in length and often results in sequences with scaffolding gaps, bias due to high GC content, repeat sequences, and missing insertions. LRS techniques produce reads between 10Kb and 40Kb [24–27].

Illumina is the dominant SRS platform by supporting paired-end sequencing (although other platforms exist including Thermo Fisher Scientific, Ion Torrent, and Complete Genomics) [28], whereas Pacific Biosystems and Oxford Nanopore Technologies sequencers are dominant in generating long reads. There are several advantages SRS have which include high throughput, low cost per base, and a low raw read rate [28]. However, the short-read length complicates genome alignment leading to false-positive and false-negative variant calling [29, 30]. Furthermore, *de novo* assembly of short sequencing reads can be challenging due to minimal overlap between raw reads, which therefore require enhanced algorithms for successful assembly, such as SOAPdenovo [31], in order to assemble a large genome of interest, although genome assemblies, especially for non-model organisms, generated from SRS are limited as long-range linking information is limited [32].

There are several variant algorithm detection methods, including FreeBayes [33] that are specific for SRS data. The advantages for SRS for MRD include low error rate and the ability to generate deep coverage for a specific region of the genome. Therefore, SRS has dominated the field for cancer genomics as variant detection is more accurate with SRS over LRS techniques that have a higher error rate and less sensitive limit of detection.

More than 70% of genetic variations seen in humans are non-SNP variations and can be missed easily with short-read sequencing [34]. Long-read sequencing enables reads longer than 10 kb, which improves alignment to the reference genome, high consensus accuracy, uniform coverage, and detection of epigenetic modifications. In addition, long-read sequencing is beneficial in transcriptomic analyses as it allows detection of splice isoforms with a high level of confidence without requiring assembly. High costs of long-read sequencing and high error rates are the major hurdle for adopting these platforms as a global sequencing platform.

Roche 454 Pyrosequencing

The first commercially available second-generation sequencer was developed by 454 Life Sciences in 2005 and was based on pyrosequencing. In 2007, 454 Life Sciences was acquired by Roche [24]. Pyrosequencing is based on the detection of light signal generated by the release of pyrophosphate (PPi) upon incorporation of dNTP in presence of ATP sulfurylase, luciferase, DNA polymerase, and adenosine 5′-phosphosulfate (APS). Luciferase ATP mediates conversion of luciferin to oxyluciferin, which generates a light signal during repeated nucleotide incorporation into the newly synthesized DNA chain. The ability to run massive sequencing reactions in parallel per run is the obvious advantage of this machine. DNA libraries were tagged to beads using adaptor sequences and using emulsion PCR in a pico-liter plate where ideally each well gets one DNA bead [23]. This miniaturized system used massively parallelized sequencing to produce more than 200,000 reads at 100–150 bp per read with an output of 20 Mb per run in 2005 [35].

In 2008, Roche released the new version 454 GS FLX titanium system with improved average read length up to 700 bp with an accuracy of 99.997% and an output of 0.7 Gb of data per run within 24 h. Roche combined the 454 sequencing system in 2009 with the GS junior, a benchtop system. This new application simplified library preparation protocol, improved data processing steps, and improved the time requirements per run to 14 h. The use of these systems was limited by the high cost of reagents and high error rates in homopolymer repeats [26, 36–38]. However, with the commercial availability of the sequencing, various other companies have launched new sequencers as discussed below.

Illumina (Solexa) Sequencers

In 2006, Solexa released the Genome Analyzer (GA), and in 2007 the company was purchased by Illumina. The Illumina sequencer is different from the Roche 454 sequencer as it uses bridge amplification for colony generation and is based on the sequencing by synthesis (SBS) approach. The library with fixed adaptors is denatured to single strands and grafted to a flow cell, followed by bridge amplification to form clusters (miniature colonies or polonies) that contain clonal DNA fragments. Sequencing by synthesis approach uses removable fluorescently labeled chain-terminating nucleotides, which produce a larger output at lower reagent cost. All the steps during sequencing in the Illumina technology are carried out in a flow cell. Flow cells can have single or multiple lanes depending upon the Illumina instrument.

Illumina provides two styles of sequencing machines – benchtop sequencers (MiniSeq System, MiSeq Series, and NextSeq Series) and production scale sequencers (NextSeq Series, HiSeq Series, HiSeq X Series, and NovaSeq 600 system). These sequencers range from low (0.3Gb) to mid (120Gb) and to high output (1500 Gb). In the present day, Illumina is the dominant sequencing platform for clinical research efforts.

Sequencing by Oligonucleotide Ligation and Detection (SOLiD)

Supported oligonucleotide ligation and detection (SOLiD) is another next-generation application that was first released in 2008 by Applied Biosystems Instruments (ABI) and marketed by Life Technologies. This platform is based on two-nucleotide sequencing by ligation (SBL) strategy where sequential annealing of probes is followed by ligation. This process generates hundreds of millions to billions of short reads with simultaneous two-base encoding for each nucleotide. Sequencer 5500 W series with either one (5500 W system) or two (5500xl system) flow chips are present in the market which are suitable for small- and large-scale projects involving whole genomes, exomes, small RNA, and transcriptomes [39]. As each base is interrogated twice, this platform provides a high accuracy of 99.85% after filtering in addition to the low cost per base; however, short-read lengths (35–85 bp), long run times (7–14 days), and requirement of huge computational infrastructure are major shortcomings [17, 40].

Ion Torrent

The Ion Torrent technology is another platform produced by the inventors of 454 sequencing [41]. This technology is fundamentally different from other platforms as it does not use either fluorescence or luminescence (post-light sequencing technology) but instead uses microchip amalgamated flow cells coupled with electronic sensors. The incorporation of a single nucleotide releases a proton which results in a change of pH and can be measured electronically as a voltage change; if there are two nucleotides added, double voltage is detected [17]. Two sequencing platforms, Proton Sequencer (with more than 165 million sensors) and the Ion Personal Genome Machine (PGM) (a benchtop sequencer with 11.1 million sensors), adapted this technology. Of interest, this technique does not require fluorescence. and the utilization of camera scanning improves the speed, cost, and size of the instrument. The major disadvantages include short-read length and problem in reading homopolymer stretches and repeats [4, 38].

DNA Nanoball Sequencing (DNBS)

DNA nanoball sequencing (DNBS) was developed by the inventor of SBH as a hybrid sequencing application that uses hybridization and ligation. Using four adapter sequences, small fragments of genomic DNA or cDNA (400–500 bp) are amplified into microscopic DNA nanoballs (roughly 300 nm in size) by rolling circle amplification, generating ssDNA concatemer. The DNA nanoballs are sequenced at a high density as one nanoball per well onto an arrayed flow cell. Up to ten bases of the template are read in the 5′ and 3′ direction from each adapter. Since only short sequences, adjacent to adapters, are read, this sequencing format resembles a multiplexed form of mate-pair sequencing. The short length of reads and sequencing time are the major disadvantages of DNBS, whereas the high density of arrays and therefore the high number of DNBS (~350 million) that can be sequenced are the major advantages [42].

Third-Generation Sequencing

So-called "third-generation" sequencing differs from next- (or second) generation sequencing as (i) PCR is not needed before sequencing which results in shortened time and reduced bias and error caused by PCR; (ii) the signal is captured in real time, which means that the signal, no matter whether it is fluorescent or electric current, is monitored during the enzymatic reaction of adding nucleotide in the complementary strand; (iii) it is capable of sequencing single molecule; (iv) it has low price of sequencing; and (v) it is simpler (the preparatory procedures and sequencing methods are simpler compared to second-generation sequencing).

Single-Molecule Real Time (SMRT)

Single-molecule real-time (SMRT) technology is developed by Pacific Biosciences (Menlo Park, CA, USA) and uses modified enzyme and direct observation of the enzymatic reaction in real time. SMRT cells contain 150,000 ultramicrowells where reaction takes place at a zeptoliter scale [10–21, 43]. Each well is coated with a molecule of DNA polymerase using the biotin-streptavidin system in nanostructures known as zero-mode waveguides (ZMWs) and DNA template that can be detected during the whole process.

During the reaction, fluorescently labeled dNTPs are added to the growing strand and monitored by CCD cameras.

PacBio machines produce long reads (up to and exceeding 10 kb in length), which are useful for de novo genome assemblies, and accuracy reported is >99%. Compared to other technologies, PacBio (i) adapters used in SMRT have a hairpin structure (SMRT loop adapters) which allows circularization of dsDNA after ligation and (ii) does not rely on interrupted cycles of extension and imaging to read the template strand as signals of newly added nucleotides are recorded in real time [24, 40, 43].

Helicos Sequencing

The Helicos sequencing system was the first implementation of single-molecule fluorescent sequencing. Sheared DNA is tailed with polyA tail and hybridized in a flow cell surface coated with oligo-dT for sequencing by synthesis of billions of molecules in parallel. The fluorescent signals were used to detect labeled nucleotide triphosphates incorporated onto DNA templates bound to a quartz slide. This technology sequences the DNA by both the hybridization and sequencing by synthesis using a DNA polymerase. The HeliScope sequencing read lengths range from 25 to over 60 bases, with 35 bases being the average. The Seqll (http://seqll.com) markets this technology to sequences genomic DNA and RNA using the Helicos sequencing system and HeliScope single-molecule sequencers. This method has successfully sequenced the human genome and provided disease signatures in a clinical evaluation and was implemented for sequencing RNA molecules for quantitative transcriptomic analysis of tissues and cells [44–46].

Next-Generation Sequencing by Electron Microscopy

Though detection is not easy, electron microscopy allows the direct visualization of the sequence of DNA molecules. Samples were sequenced by the enzymatic incorporation of modified bases with atoms of increased atomic number.

These high atomic number atoms allow the direct visualization and identification of individually labeled bases under the electron microscope as dark dots. Direct visualization and identification of individually labeled bases within a synthetic 3272 base-pair DNA molecule and a 7249 base-pair viral genome have been demonstrated [47, 48]; however, the technology has not yet been commercially developed.

Two companies, ZS Genetics (http://www.zsgenetics.com) and Electron Optica [49], are continuously working on the DNA sequencing technique by electron microscopy, with different approaches. ZS Genetics demonstrated the labeling and identification of the four bases of DNA with an electron microscopy for the first time in the year 2012. The sequence read lengths range from 5 to 50 kb and are useful for de novo genome assembly and for analysis of full haplotypes and copy number variants (http://www.zsgenetics.com).

However, the heavy atom labeling has few disadvantages which include: (i) chances of incomplete labeling reaction which might result in missing few base pairs, (ii) four different reactions have to run as the labels are difficult to distinguish and interfere with each other when they get too close, and (iii) high-energy electrons damage the DNA and therefore cause errors to precisely locate the bases [47, 50]. Electron Optica uses low-energy electron microscopy (LEEM) which does not need labeling with heavy metals for DNA sequencing. Though LEEM causes less damage to DNA and thus reduces sequencing errors [48, 51, 52], there is no update on this technology since 2014 [49].

Fourth-Generation Sequencing

The fourth-generation sequencing platforms sequence without amplification, real-time sequencing without repeated cycles, and elimination of synthesis. These technologies preserve the spatial coordinates of DNA and RNA sequences with up to subcellular resolution, thus enabling back mapping of sequencing reads to the original histological context [22, 27].

Nanopore Sequencing

Nanopore-based sequencers open a new door to molecular biology investigation at the single-molecule scale. In the 1990s, Church et al. and Deamer and Akeson separately proposed sequencing of DNA using nanopores [53, 54]. The sequencing of DNA is done by passing the single-stranded DNA molecule through a nanopore chamber, which can be found in protein channel which facilitates ion exchange. With the application of an external voltage, particles with sizes smaller than the pore size are passed through the pore which are either embedded in a biological membrane or formed in solid-state film. Major advantages include simple experimental procedure, required no labeling and less input, and generate real-time data with ultra-long reads and high throughput [4, 53, 55]. The nanopore sequencer has wider applications in many areas, such as analysis of DNA, RNA, proteins, peptides, drugs, polymers, etc. [4, 55, 56].

The nanopores can either be from the biological system or solid-state synthetic nanopores. In combination with the other devices and electronic circuits, these pores are integrated in a form of portable sequencing chips. Biological nanopores, also termed transmembrane protein channels, are usually embedded in liposomes or polymer films. There are three main biological experiments involving this technology and the study of *Staphylococcus aureus* α hemolysin (α HL), *Mycobacterium smegmatis* porin A (MspA), and *Bacteriophage* phi29. On the other hand, solid-state synthetic systems fabricate nanopores in silicon nitride (Si_3N_4), silicon dioxide (SiO_2), aluminum oxide (Al_2O_3), boron nitride (BN), graphene, polymer membranes, and hybrid materials [4, 17, 53, 55].

Solid-state nanopore is reliably more stable than biological and could be multiplexed to work in parallel on a single device and achieve higher readout within a short time. Oxford Nanopore Technologies (ONT) (https://nanoporetech.com), founded by Hagan Bayley and Gordon Sanghera, provide the commercially available nanopore sequencing instruments that provide real-time data. Major devices from ONT include MinION (pocket-sized, portable device), GridIONX5 (multiplex sequencing device), PromethION (high-throughput, high-sample number benchtop system), and SmidgION (smallest device designed for use with a smartphone in any location) (https://nanoporetech.com). One of the major disadvantages of this technology is the rapid DNA translocation velocity (1–3 ls/base) which limits the identification of single nucleotide bases and increases error rate (up to 90%) [57].

Success with this platform has been noted by combining results with short-read sequencing to improve error rates at the single-base resolution while also producing reads long enough for de novo assembly efforts [58]. Using this technique Goodwin et al. were able to create an open-source hybrid error correction algorithm, Nanocorr, that combines Illumina SRS (MiSeq) data and Nanopore, which enhanced genome assembly and variant detection [59].

BioNano Genomics

BioNano's next-generation mapping uses nano-channel arrays with optical mapping to image extremely long, high-molecular-weight DNA in its most native state instead of classical DNA sequencing devices. This technology provides a detailed genome map, which helps to finish sequencing and to remove sequencing errors caused by repetitive regions. Genome map in addition to the sequencing provides a better resolution of the whole genome, showing its features in context and functional relationships, across kilobases to megabases. BioNano Saphyr provides rapid, high-throughput, long-range genome mapping with the ability to detect the large-scale structural variations (ranging from 1 kb to megabases) missed by next-generation sequencing (NGS) systems (https://bionanogenomics.com/products/saphyr/). The high-resolution Irys System from BioNano Genomics offers whole-genome maps at a single-molecule resolution.

Emerging Platforms: Single-Cell Sequencing (SCS)

Advancements in microfluidics have enabled the robust isolation of single cells, which then facilitates individual cellular analysis of DNA or RNA. Bulk sequencing analyses are based on an averaged signal obtained from a heterogeneous cell or nucleic acid population and therefore obviate resolution at a cellular level – which is overcome via single-cell analysis [60, 61]. Single-cell sequencing is rapidly becoming established as an important tool in a diverse series of disciplines ranging from characterization of cellular diversity to identification of new cell types [62, 63]. Over the past decade, there has been extraordinary progress in the development and application of single-cell DNA and RNA sequencing methods. Studies by Tang et al. (2009) [64] and Navin et al. (2011) [60] describing single-cell RNA and DNA analysis, respectively, are pioneering discoveries in the field. As we are moving toward the era of precision medicine, the data generated from multiple "omics" strategies provides complex insight on biological events. Single-cell analyses of DNA, RNA, and protein generate data demonstrating the heterogeneity of a given cellular network, which ultimately leads to improved understanding of the underlying mechanisms of any physiologic or disease-related process. Every improvement in these assays increases sensitivity and throughput. Additional applications in which single-cell sequencing could offer new insights are with respect to circulating tumor cells prior to a diagnosis, residual circulating cancer cells post-therapy, and stem cell identification and specification. Single-cell arrays provide tools to measure different aspects of various substrates (like DNA for chromatin structure, histone modification, or sequence variability; RNA for gene expression changes, allele-specific expression, fusion events; protein for correlating surface immunophenotypes or ligand-receptor interactions, and many others) [60, 61, 65]. These platforms are expanding rapidly (Table 1.1), and single-cell RNA sequencing platforms have been reviewed elsewhere [66].

Each platform possesses its own unique profile of advantages and disadvantages depending upon the intended application.

In conclusion, the ultimate goal of true precision (personalized) therapy for cancer or several other diseases rests on the accurate characterization of the systemic heterogeneity in genetic and epigenetic variability combined with understanding their respective and additive impact on cellular function as it relates to risk prognostication and therapeutic selection. MRD is a direct reflection of how biomedical scientists and clinicians have applied exciting new technologies to understand the minutiae of human physiology in order to improve human health.

TABLE 1.1 Overview of currently available single-cell sequencing platforms

Method or company	Applications and references
Drop-Seq	RNA-Seq [67]
InDrops	RNA-Seq [68]
CEL-Seq2	RNA-Seq [69]
Quartz-Seq2	RNA-Seq [70]
Cyto-Seq	RNA-Seq [71]
MARS-Seq	RNA-Seq [72]
Hi-SCL	RNA-Seq [73]
Chromium System (10x Genomics)	RNA-Seq, DNA-Seq, immune repertoire profiling
Nadia (Dolomite Bio)	RNA-Seq, DNA-Seq
ddSEQ Single-Cell Isolator (Bio-Rad)	RNA-Seq
Tapestri Platform (MissionBio)	Targeted DNA-Seq
BD Rhapsody Single-Cell Analysis System (Becton Dickinson)	Targeted RNA-Seq
C1 System and Polaris (Fluidigm)	RNA-Seq, DNA-Seq, miRNA-Seq, epigenomics, RT-qPCR

References

1. Young AL, Challen GA, Birmann BM, et al. Clonal haematopoiesis harbouring AML-associated mutations is ubiquitous in healthy adults. Nat Commun. 2016;7:12484.
2. The History of DNA Timeline, https://www.dna-worldwide.com/resource/160/history-dna-timeline.
3. Holley RW, Apgar J, Everett GA, et al. Structure of a ribonucleic acid. Science. 1965;147:1462–5.
4. Buermans HPJ, den Dunnen JT. Next generation sequencing technology: advances and applications. Biochim Biophys Acta BBA Mol Basis Dis. 2014;1842:1932–41.
5. Heather JM, Chain B. The sequence of sequencers: the history of sequencing DNA. Genomics. 2016;107:1–8.
6. Sanger F, Brownlee GG, Barrell BG. A two-dimensional fractionation procedure for radioactive nucleotides. J Mol Biol. 1965;13:373–98.
7. Wu R, Kaiser AD. Structure and base sequence in the cohesive ends of bacteriophage lambda DNA. J Mol Biol. 1968;35:523–37.
8. Jou WM, Haegeman G, Ysebaert M, et al. Nucleotide sequence of the gene coding for the bacteriophage MS2 coat protein. Nature. 1972;237:82.
9. Fiers W, Contreras R, Duerinck F, et al. Complete nucleotide sequence of bacteriophage MS2 RNA: primary and secondary structure of the replicase gene. Nature. 1976;260:500.
10. Sanger F, Coulson AR. A rapid method for determining sequences in DNA by primed synthesis with DNA polymerase. J Mol Biol. 1975;94:441–8.
11. Sanger F, Air GM, Barrell BG, et al. Nucleotide sequence of bacteriophage φX174 DNA. Nature. 1977;265:687.
12. Maxam AM, Gilbert W. A new method for sequencing DNA. Proc Natl Acad Sci U S A. 1977;74:560–4.
13. Smith LM, Sanders JZ, Kaiser RJ, et al. Fluorescence detection in automated DNA sequence analysis. Nature. 1986;321:674.
14. Anderson S. Shotgun DNA sequencing using cloned DNase I-generated fragments. Nucleic Acids Res. 1981;9:3015–27.
15. Ansorge WJ. Next-generation DNA sequencing techniques. New Biotechnol. 2009;25:195–203.
16. Adams MD, Kelley JM, Gocayne JD, et al. Complementary DNA sequencing: expressed sequence tags and human genome project. Science. 1991;252:1651–6.

17. Kulski JK. Next-generation sequencing — an overview of the history, tools, and "Omic" applications: InTech; 2016. http://creativecommons.org/licenses/by/3.0.
18. Bumgarner R. DNA microarrays: types, applications and their future. Curr Protoc Mol Biol Ed Frederick M Ausubel Al. 2013;0 22:Unit-22.1.
19. Fleischmann RD, Adams MD, White O, et al. Whole-genome random sequencing and assembly of haemophilus influenzae Rd. Science. 1995;269:496–512.
20. Fraser CM, Gocayne JD, White O, et al. The minimal gene complement of mycoplasma genitalium. Science. 1995;270:397–404.
21. Stein L. Genome annotation: from sequence to biology. Nat Rev Genet. 2001;2:493.
22. Ke R, Mignardi M, Hauling T, et al. Fourth generation of next-generation sequencing technologies: promise and consequences. Hum Mutat. 2016;37:1363–7.
23. Koboldt DC, Steinberg KM, Larson DE, et al. The next-generation sequencing revolution and its impact on genomics. Cell. 2013;155:27–38.
24. Liu L, Li Y, Li S, et al. Comparison of next-generation sequencing systems, https://www.hindawi.com/journals/bmri/2012/251364/.
25. Illumina | Sequencing and array-based solutions for genetic research, https://www.illumina.com/index-d.html.
26. SE L, Myers RM. Advancements in next-generation sequencing. Annu Rev Genomics Hum Genet. 2016;17:95–115.
27. Srinivasan S, Batra J. Four generations of sequencing- is it ready for the clinic yet? J Gener Seq Appl. 2014;1:107.
28. Caspar SM, Dubacher N, Kopps AM, et al. Clinical sequencing: from raw data to diagnosis with lifetime value. Clin Genet:n/a–a.
29. Derrien T, Estellé J, Sola SM, et al. Fast computation and applications of genome Mappability. PLoS One. 2012;7:e30377.
30. Mandelker D, Schmidt RJ, Ankala A, et al. Navigating highly homologous genes in a molecular diagnostic setting: a resource for clinical next-generation sequencing. Genet Med. 2016;18:1282.
31. Li R, Zhu H, Ruan J, et al. De novo assembly of human genomes with massively parallel short read sequencing. Genome Res. 2010;20:265–72.
32. The Long and the Short of DNA Sequencing, https://www.genengnews.com/gen-exclusives/the-long-and-the-short-of-dna-sequencing/77899725.
33. Garrison E, Marth G. Haplotype-based variant detection from short-read sequencing. arXiv preprint arXiv. 2012;1207.3907 [q-bio.GN].

34. The 1000 Genomes Project Consortium. A map of human genome variation from population scale sequencing. Nature. 2010;467:1061–73.
35. van Dijk EL, Auger H, Jaszczyszyn Y, et al. Ten years of next-generation sequencing technology. Trends Genet. 2014;30:418–26.
36. Bio-IT World, http://www.bio-itworld.com.
37. Yuzuki D. Next-generation sequencing - its historical context, 2012, http://www.yuzuki.org/next-generation-sequencing-its-historical-context/
38. Yohe S, Thyagarajan B. Review of clinical next-generation sequencing. Arch Pathol Lab Med. 2017;141:1544–57.
39. SOLiD® Next-Generation Sequencing Systems & Accessories, https://www.thermofisher.com/us/en/home/life-science/sequencing/next-generation-sequencing/solid-next-generation-sequencing/solid-next-generation-sequencing-systems-reagents-accessories.html.
40. Kruglyak KM, Lin E, Ong FS. Next-generation sequencing and applications to the diagnosis and treatment of lung Cancer. Adv Exp Med Biol. 2016;890:123–36.
41. Rothberg JM, Hinz W, Rearick TM, et al. An integrated semiconductor device enabling non-optical genome sequencing. Nature. 2011;475:348.
42. Human Genome Sequencing Using Unchained Base Reads on Self-Assembling DNA Nanoarrays | Science, http://science.sciencemag.org/content/327/5961/78.long.
43. Koren S, Harhay GP, Smith TP, et al. Reducing assembly complexity of microbial genomes with single-molecule sequencing. Genome Biol. 2013;14:R101.
44. Thompson JF, Steinmann KE. Single molecule sequencing with a HeliScope genetic analysis system. In: Current protocols in molecular biology. Hoboken: Wiley; 2001.
45. Ashley EA, Butte AJ, Wheeler MT, et al. Clinical assessment incorporating a personal genome. Lancet. 2010;375:1525–35.
46. Hickman SE, Kingery ND, Ohsumi TK, et al. The microglial sensome revealed by direct RNA sequencing. Nat Neurosci. 2013;16:1896.
47. Bell DC, Thomas WK, Murtagh KM, et al. DNA Base identification by Electron microscopy. Microsc Microanal. 2012;18:1049–53.
48. Mankos M, Shadman K, Persson HHJ, et al. A novel low energy electron microscope for DNA sequencing and surface analysis. Ultramicroscopy. 2014;145:36–49.

49. NEWS, http://www.electronoptica.com/Electron_optica/NEWS.html.
50. Ari Ş, Arikan M. Next-generation sequencing: advantages, disadvantages, and future, in: plant Omics: trends and applications. Cham: Springer; 2016. p. 109–35.
51. Mankos M, Shadman K, N'Diaye AT, et al. Progress toward an aberration-corrected low energy electron microscope for DNA sequencing and surface analysis. J Vac Sci Technol B Nanotechnol Microelectron. 2012;30:6F402.
52. Mankos M, Persson HHJ, N'Diaye AT, et al. Nucleotide-specific contrast for DNA sequencing by Electron spectroscopy. PLoS One. 2016;11:e0154707.
53. Deamer DW, Akeson M. Nanopores and nucleic acids: prospects for ultrarapid sequencing. Trends Biotechnol. 2000;18:147–51.
54. Feng Y, Zhang Y, Ying C, et al. Nanopore-based fourth-generation DNA sequencing technology. Genomics Proteomics Bioinformatics. 2015;13:4–16.
55. Ansorge WJ. Next generation DNA sequencing (II): techniques, applications. Next Generat Sequenc & Applic. 2016;S1:005. https://doi.org/10.4172/2469-9853.S1-005.
56. Jain M, Olsen HE, Paten B, et al. The Oxford Nanopore MinION: delivery of nanopore sequencing to the genomics community. Genome Biol. 2016;17:239.
57. Mikheyev AS, Tin MMY. A first look at the Oxford Nanopore MinION sequencer. Mol Ecol Resour. 2014;14:1097–102.
58. Laver T, Harrison J, O'Neill PA, et al. Assessing the performance of the Oxford Nanopore technologies MinION. Biomol Detect Quantif. 2015;3:1–8.
59. Goodwin S, Gurtowski J, Ethe-Sayers S, et al. Oxford Nanopore sequencing, hybrid error correction, and de novo assembly of a eukaryotic genome. Genome Res. 2015;25:1750–6.
60. Navin N, Kendall J, Troge J, et al. Tumour evolution inferred by single-cell sequencing. Nature. 2011;472:90–4.
61. Gawad C, Koh W, Quake SR. Single-cell genome sequencing: current state of the science. Nat Rev Genet. 2016;17:175–88.
62. Kester L, van Oudenaarden A. Single-cell Transcriptomics meets lineage tracing. Cell Stem Cell. 2018;23(2):166–79.
63. Ortega MA, Poirion O, Zhu X, et al. Using single-cell multiple omics approaches to resolve tumor heterogeneity. Clin Transl Med. 2017;6(46):46.

64. Tang F, Barbacioru C, Wang Y, et al. mRNA-Seq whole-transcriptome analysis of a single cell. Nat Methods. 2009;6:377–82.
65. Wang Y, Navin NE. Advances and applications of single-cell sequencing technologies. Mol Cell. 2015;58:598–609.
66. Picelli S. Single-cell RNA-sequencing: the future of genome biology is now. RNA Biol. 2017;14:637–50.
67. Macosko EZ, Basu A, Satija R, et al. Highly parallel genome-wide expression profiling of individual cells using Nanoliter droplets. Cell. 2015;161:1202–14.
68. Klein AM, Mazutis L, Akartuna I, et al. Droplet barcoding for single-cell Transcriptomics applied to embryonic stem cells. Cell. 2015;161:1187–201.
69. Hashimshony T, Senderovich N, Avital G, et al. CEL-Seq2: sensitive highly-multiplexed single-cell RNA-Seq. Genome Biol. 2016;17(77):77.
70. Sasagawa Y, Danno H, Takada H, et al. Quartz-Seq2: a high-throughput single-cell RNA-sequencing method that effectively uses limited sequence reads. Genome Biol. 2018;19:29.
71. Fan HC, Fu GK, Fodor SPA. Combinatorial labeling of single cells for gene expression cytometry. Science. 2015;347:1258367.
72. Jaitin DA, Kenigsberg E, Keren-Shaul H, et al. Massively parallel single-cell RNA-Seq for marker-free decomposition of tissues into cell types. Science. 2014;343:776–9.
73. Rotem A, Ram O, Shoresh N, et al. High-throughput single-cell labeling (hi-SCL) for RNA-Seq using drop-based microfluidics. PLoS One. 2015;10:e0116328.

Chapter 2
Minimal Residual Disease Testing in Acute Lymphoblastic Leukemia/Lymphoma

Laura Wake, Xueyan Chen, and Michael J. Borowitz

Introduction

Acute lymphoblastic leukemia (ALL) is a clonal hematopoietic stem cell disorder of precursor B or T lymphocytes presenting as undifferentiated-appearing lymphoblasts in the bone marrow, peripheral blood, or extramedullary tissue. While it is a rare disease overall, it is the most common malignancy in the pediatric age group, with B-ALL affecting 4–5/100,000 children per year [1]. T-ALL is less common than B-ALL, comprising 10–15% of childhood ALL and 25% of adult ALL, although T-lymphoblastic lymphoma (LBL) is much more common than B-LBL, comprising 85–90% of all LBLs [1, 2].

L. Wake · M. J. Borowitz (✉)
Department of Pathology, Johns Hopkins Medical Institutions, Baltimore, MD, USA
e-mail: mborowitz@jhmi.edu

X. Chen
Department of Pathology, University of Washington, Seattle, WA, USA

Current intensive chemotherapeutic treatment regimens, including induction, consolidation, and maintenance therapy, are highly effective in ALL. The 5-year disease-free survival (DFS) in pediatric B-ALL patients is >85% for most risk groups, and the cure rate is >90% [3–5]. The prognosis has also improved for patients with T-ALL over the last 20 years, from a 5-year event-free survival (EFS) in children of 75% to currently >90% [6, 7].

Despite these favorable statistics, a subset of patients has unfavorable risk factors, a greater chance of relapse, and therefore worse overall prognosis. In 1993, a National Cancer Institute (NCI) workshop defined and standardized risk criteria for pediatric B-ALL for prognostic purposes [8]. The two main identifiable risk factors for B-ALL at that time were age and WBC count, followed by CNS involvement, cytogenetics, DNA index (aneuploidy), and early response to treatment. These prognostic factors reliably predicted patient outcome and stratified patients into risk categories based on EFS.

Prognostic markers for T-ALL were not as well defined as in B-ALL. Early pediatric oncology group (POG) studies found that unlike B-ALL, clinical features such as older age and high WBC count were not reliable markers of outcome in patients with T-ALL [9]. However, the POG did report an association between T-lymphoblast maturation and patient outcome, a finding that was investigated by other groups, including the St. Jude Children's Research Hospital ALL 2000 trial. This study identified a subset of patients with T-ALL with genetic and immunophenotypic profiles similar to normal early thymocytes precursors (ETPs) who appeared to have higher rates of remission failure or relapse compared with non-ETP T-ALL patients (72% vs. 11%) as well as significantly worse outcomes. Recent studies, however, dispute these earlier findings and show that T-ALL patients generally have excellent outcomes, even with the ETP immunophenotype [7].

While traditional risk factors, such as age, WBC count, cytogenetics, and lymphoblastic maturation stage, are important to assess at diagnosis, none are accurate predictors of patient response and overall outcome. The most informative prognostic indicator for both B-ALL and T-ALL is response to treatment as measured by the presence or absence of residual disease after initial therapy. This measure takes into account both disease characteristics and patient characteristics, allows for future treatment planning, and is independently predictive of outcome in nearly all subgroups of patients.

Minimal Residual Disease

Rapid disease clearance during induction therapy predicts long-term outcome [10, 11]. Originally, early treatment response was evaluated by morphologic review of the bone marrow on day 14. Residual disease was categorized based on the number of blasts present, which in turn predicted EFS: M1 patients (<5% blasts) had an overall 6-year EFS of 63%; M2 (5–25% blasts) had a 6-year EFS of 44%; and M3 (>25% blasts) had a much poorer 6-year EFS of 25% [8].

However, experiments using mixtures of leukemic cells and normal cells revealed that low-level leukemic cells were not reliably detected by morphologic assessment and that a bone marrow with <5% blasts, originally considered complete remission (CR), could potentially retain up to 10^{11}–10^{12} leukemic cells as residual disease [12].

From these studies arose the concept of minimal residual disease (MRD), or disease below the morphologic level of detection, and it was soon apparent that more sophisticated methods were needed for assessing MRD status during and after treatment to quantitate the true burden of disease. Since then, numerous studies have shown the clinical significance of MRD in relation to patient prognosis, risk of relapse, and survival in B-ALL [12–19]. Specifically, MRD-positive patients have statistically significantly worse DFS and EFS, as well as increased risk of relapse (RR) and lower relapse-free survival (RFS) [12, 13, 16, 19–23]. A recent large meta-analysis encompassing more than 13,000 ALL patients from 39 published studies confirmed the association between MRD and survival and showed that MRD negativity was associated with much better 10-year EFS (77% for MRD-negative patients vs. 32% for MRD-positive patients) [24] (Fig. 2.1).

Although the precise definition of early response differs among different treatment protocols, it is now widely accepted that the presence of MRD after initial phases of therapy is the most powerful adverse predictor of outcome in children and adolescents with B-ALL [25–28]. In many studies, the presence of MRD after 4–6 weeks of therapy is used to assign patients to more intensive therapy [15, 29]. In other studies, risk stratification is dependent upon assessment of MRD at two different time points, typically after induction and consolidation therapy [20, 23, 26, 29–31]. In early studies, before MRD was used as a criterion to alter therapy, patients with MRD levels as low as 0.01% had demonstrably poorer outcome, and this level became the standard for calling a sample positive for MRD [15, 26, 27, 29] (Fig. 2.2).

Similarly, assessing MRD status is important for prognostication in patients with T-ALL, although T-ALL appears to clear from the marrow more slowly, and therefore, different thresholds are used to establish prognosis. In the large AIEOP-BFM-ALL 2000 trial, T-ALL MRD negativity at day 33 was reported as the most favorable prognostic factor, while MRD positivity at day 78 ($>10^{-3}$) was the most important predictive factor for relapse [32]. Wood et al. confirmed the significance of MRD in clinical response in T-ALL and showed day 29 MRD-positive T-ALL patients had inferior EFS and OS [7].

These studies underscore the prognostic importance of MRD status for B-ALL and T-ALL and emphasize the need for sensitive, accurate, and standardized methods of MRD detection.

Chapter 2. Minimal Residual Disease Testing in Acute 27

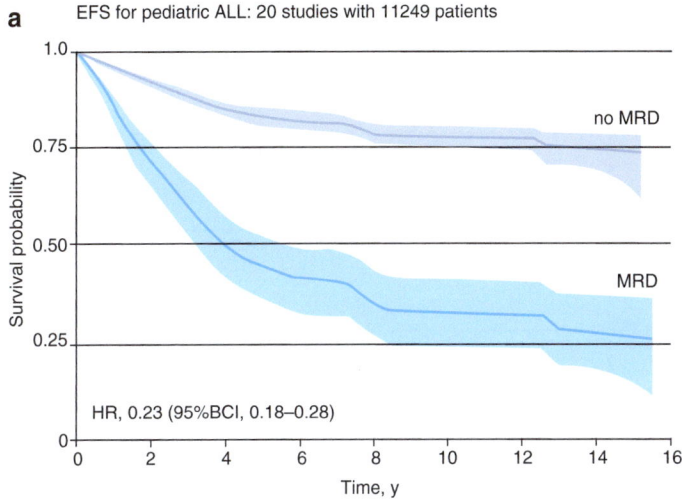

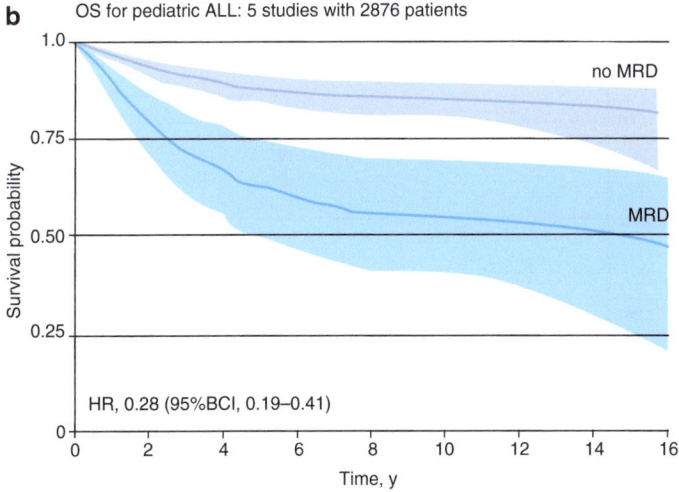

FIGURE 2.1 Event-free survival (EFS) and overall survival (OS) in ALL MRD[a]. Graphical data from a large meta-analysis of 39 published studies encompassing 13,637 ALL patients. The EFS (**a**) and OS (**b**) of pediatric patients with and without MRD, and the EFS (**c**) and OS (**d**) of adult patients with and without MRD. In all groups, patients with MRD have a statistically significantly worse EFS and OS. ([a]This research was originally published in *JAMA Oncology*. Berry et al. [24]. Reprinted by permission)

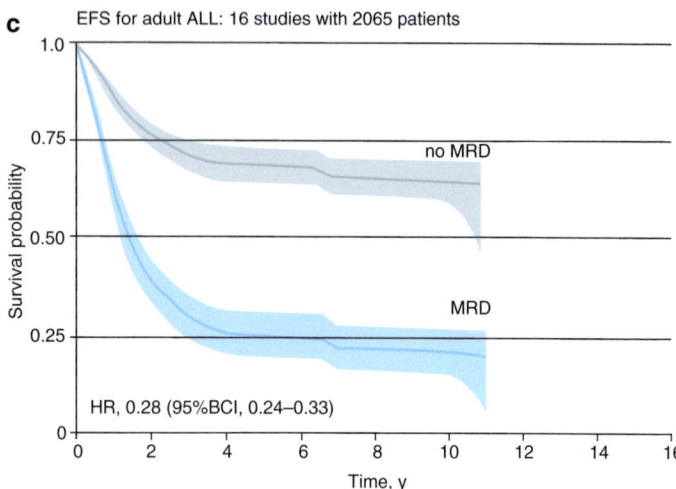

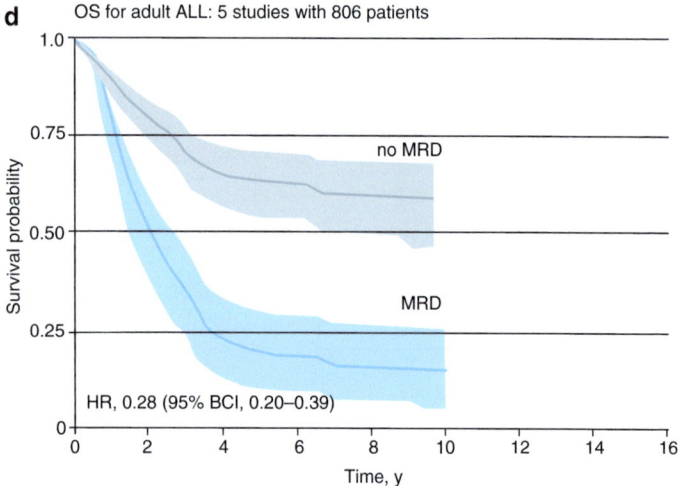

Figure 2.1 (continued)

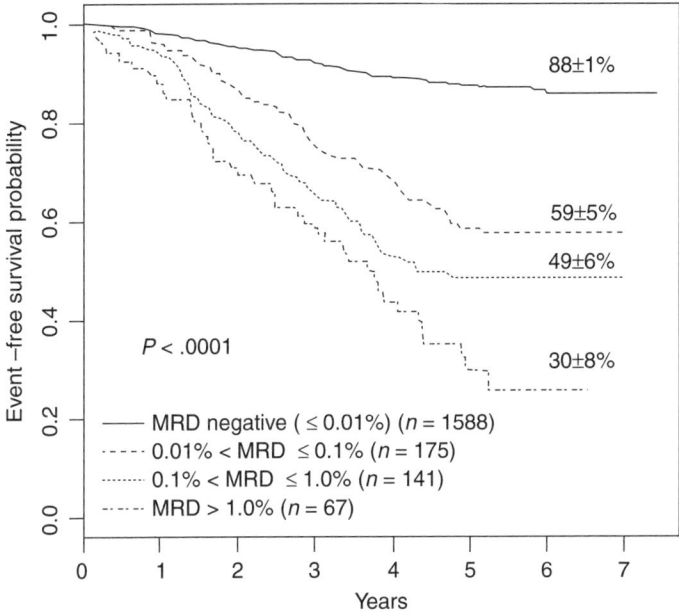

FIGURE 2.2 Event Free Survival (EFS) of patients with varying levels of MRD[a]. The 5-year EFS of patients on COG 9900 series and end-induction MRD levels. Progressively increasing MRD levels are associated with progressively worse EFS, even for those with as little as 0.01–0.1% MRD. ([a]This research was originally published in *Blood*. Borowitz et al. [28]. © The American Society of Hematology)

Methods to Assess MRD

To be useful for MRD detection, a platform must have high sensitivity, specificity, and reproducibility [11]. Morphologic assessment, even with the aid of immunohistochemical testing, lacks both sensitivity and specificity. Likewise, conventional karyotyping and florescence in situ hybridization (FISH) lacks the necessary sensitivity to detect submicroscopic leukemic cells, with levels of sensitivity approaching only 1–5% [33, 34].

Currently the main methods to assess for residual disease include flow cytometry, which depends on identifying cells with aberrant immunophenotypes, and polymerase chain reaction (PCR)-based molecular methods, directed at identifying tumor-specific sequences of antigen receptors. More recently, NGS has been used for molecular detection of these latter abnormalities (Table 2.1).

Flow Cytometry

In the earliest flow cytometric studies performed at St. Jude Children's Research Hospital, dilution experiments with leukemic cells and normal cells showed that MRD could reliably be detected at a level of one leukemic cell per 10^4 normal cells (1/10000) using a variety of well-designed antibody combinations [14]. Similarly, Weir et al., using a two-tube four-color approach, demonstrated that normal and abnormal cells could be distinguished with a similar sensitivity [35].

Detecting residual T-ALL by flow cytometry is theoretically straightforward, as the presence of any significant population of precursor T cells in the bone marrow is diagnostic. In practice, however, maturational changes, discussed further below, often make detection of specific precursor antigens problematic in the MRD setting [36], and additional detection strategies are often needed.

The major challenge in detecting residual B-ALL is distinguishing between abnormal precursor B cells and normal precursor B cells that reside and mature in the bone marrow. In the great majority of cases, leukemic precursor B-cell phenotypes differ from those of normal precursor B cells, either due to aberrant antigenic expression, loss of normal antigens, or, most commonly, abnormal expression of antigens at levels not expected for a particular stage of differentiation.

Normal B-cell precursors show precise, reproducible antigen expression during differentiation, and deviation from this pattern allows for recognition of MRD [35, 37] (Fig. 2.3). With relatively simple antibody panels, 95–98% of patients

TABLE 2.1 Methodologies of MRD detection

Method	Sensitivity	Target	Specimen	TAT	Cost	Availability	Advantage	Disadvantage
Conventional karyotype	1–5%	Numerical or structural chromosomal abnormalities	Fresh, viable cells	7–10 days	Less expensive	Widely available	Standard technique Direct quantitation	Limited sensitivity Requires metaphase cells Laborious
FISH	0.3–5%	Gene deletion, amplification, or fusion	DNA	7–10 days	Less expensive	Widely available	Rapid Standard technique Direct quantitation	Limited sensitivity Limited applicability (only detects chromosomal abnormalities)
mFC	3–4 colors, 0.1–0.01% 6–10 colors, 0.01–0.001%	LAIPs Difference from viable normal	Fresh, cells	1–2 days	Moderately expensive	Widely available	Rapid Direct quantitation ID and monitor treatment	Requires expertise May misdiagnose immunophenotypic shifts or regenerating blasts

(continued)

TABLE 2.1 (continued)

Method	Sensitivity	Target	Specimen	TAT	Cost	Availability	Advantage	Disadvantage
qPCR	0.01–0.001%	IGH/TCR gene rearrangements	DNA	4 weeks to generate patient-specific primers	More expensive	Widely available	Highly sensitive Standardized	High cost Time-consuming Laborious Requires prior knowledge of mutation status for rearrangements May miss clonal evolutions
RT-PCR	0.01–0.001%	Fusion transcripts	RNA	1–3 days	Moderately expensive	Widely available	Rapid Highly sensitive	Limited applicability (only detects leukemic cells with fusion proteins)
NGS	0.0001%	Mutated genes	DNA	1–2 weeks	Most expensive	Mostly experimental	Highly sensitive Can detect clonal evolution	High cost Time-consuming Requires prior knowledge of mutation status for rearrangements

Adapted from Chen and Wood [90]. © The American Society of Hematology. Reprinted by permission

Abbreviations: *TAT* Turn-around-time, *FISH* florescence in situ hybridization, *mFC* multiparametric flow cytometry, *qPCR* quantitative polymerase chain reaction, *RT-PCT* reverse transcriptase PCR, *NGS* next generation sequencing, *LAIPs* leukemic-associated immunophenotypes, *IGH* immunoglobulin heavy chain, *TCR* T-cell receptor

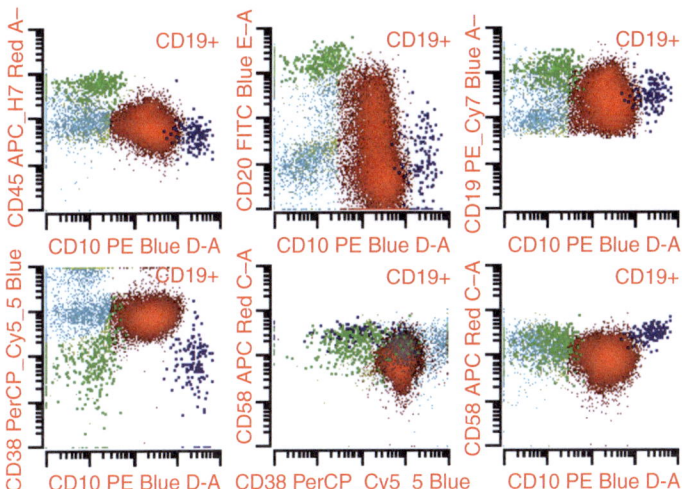

FIGURE 2.3 Normal B-cell maturation pattern with abnormal population. Using appropriate antibody combinations, flow cytometry can detect normal B-cell precursors by distinct patterns of maturation and can identify residual leukemia blasts by deviation from this pattern. In this plot of CD19-gated bone marrow, the leukemic blasts (blue) are identified by their abnormal expression of bright CD10 and CD58 with relative loss of CD38. Mature B cells are in green, normal precursor B cells in red, and plasma cells and plasmablasts in cyan

have ALL immunophenotypes that are sufficiently different from normal to detect MRD at a level of sensitivity of 0.01% [14, 28] early in therapy when marrow regeneration of normal B-precursors is limited. However, in the presence of large numbers of regenerating hematogones, more extensive panels may be necessary to detect all cases, and it may be more difficult to achieve a level of sensitivity of 1/10000.

Phenotypic Switch and Drug-Induced Immunophenotypic Modulation

Many early flow cytometric immunophenotyping studies used panels of antibodies at diagnosis to characterize abnormalities, often referred to as leukemia-associated immunophenotypes (LAIPs). Abnormal lymphoblasts with LAIPs can be detected occupying distinct regions on dual parameter displays in regions where no normal cells reside. After therapy, patient samples are reassessed for the presence of cells in these predefined areas, which indicates residual disease. Notably, this approach of MRD detection relies on the prerequisite knowledge of the diagnostic ALL immunophenotype.

While most patients continue to have LAIP after treatment, antigenic expression on the leukemic clone may change over time and/or with therapy which may result in false negatives [11, 38]. These phenotypic shifts are usually only problematic for "fixed-gate" approaches to MRD detection, in which the gating technique only assesses populations in a predefined area, and with the diagnostic phenotype. However, in general, phenotypic changes are not a major source of false negatives in flow cytometric MRD testing if one does not use a fixed-gate approach.

Most of the phenotypic changes that occur produce phenotypes that are sufficiently different from normal B cells to permit their detection (see below). Moreover, many phenotypic changes are transient. In one study, Borowitz et al. showed that although 69% of B-ALLs had a significant change in phenotype between diagnosis and relapse, the majority of MRD phenotypes resembled the diagnostic phenotype, while only 27% had an MRD phenotype that resembled the relapse specimen [39].

Many changes in phenotype are related to therapy, particularly steroid treatment. These changes occur in both the blast population and in normal precursor B cells [40, 41] and typically include down-modulation of CD10 and CD34 expressions and up-modulation of CD20 and CD45 expressions, while CD58, CD38, and CD19 usually remain stable. But because of these changes, the preferred method of MRD detection by flow cytometry is a "different from normal" approach. Although knowledge of the diagnostic ALL immunophenotype can be helpful, this approach does not depend on it. However, it does require that individuals performing and interpreting flow cytometry have expert knowledge of normal patterns of cellular maturation and, in the case of T-cell MRD analysis, familiarity with the normal presence of small populations of unusual T and NK cells. Using standard panels with this approach allows technologists and pathologists to become familiar with normal maturation patterns associated with particular antibody combinations [35, 37, 38, 42].

Flow Cytometry Panels

To aid in detecting B-ALL MRD, many authors recommended using a combination of flow cytometric panels [12, 38, 43–47]. Using more antigens prevents both false negatives due to antigenic shifts and false positives by more clearly defining normal B-cell precursors.

Early studies of B-ALL MRD detection used three-color antibody-fluorescent conjugates, with antibodies to CD19, CD10, and CD34, which were shown to be a particularly effective combination to use in the peripheral blood. In several studies, four-color flow panels were utilized, and in a study from the Children's Oncology Group (COG), a two-tube four-color panel was sufficient to identify aberrant phenotypes in >90% of patients for disease monitoring, while the other 10% of cases required additional markers [48, 49]. This panel was useful in risk-stratifying patients by MRD levels at the end of induction. With the advent of tandem dyes, six-, eight-, and even ten- or more-color panels have been used for MRD studies in ALL. In COG studies, a two-tube six-color panel compared favorably to the historical four-color panel [29], and several studies have advocated for single-tube eight-color approaches, as they have been shown to be more efficient without losing diagnostic power [47].

Although using more colors may be more efficient, especially in samples with limited cells, as of yet, there are no definitive studies which demonstrate that more colors per se allow detection of MRD that cannot be detected with smaller panels. In addition, the use of additional colors must be weighed against the training and validation needed to adopt such complex panels [11, 38, 46, 50].

Thus, choosing a flow cytometry panel for ALL is subjective. Any method chosen must be able to achieve a sensitivity of at least 1/10000 cells. The sensitivity of a test depends not only on the number of cells acquired but also, most importantly, on the degree of difference of the phenotype of the leukemic cells from any normal mature or immature B cells in the specimen. This latter problem, coupled with the expert knowledge required to make these distinctions, has made it difficult to define a single optimal panel. Nevertheless, there is a growing consensus regarding the most important markers to be part of any panel used for MRD detection (Table 2.2). In addition, an ideal panel should comprise reagents that are stable and with patterns of spectral overlap that avoid compromising the ability to detect crucial antigens. Finally, gating strategies must be relatively straightforward to allow technologists and pathologists to learn to demonstrate abnormal populations.

Molecular PCR

In the 1980–1990s, molecular PCR was investigated as a tool to evaluate residual ALL. PCR can evaluate MRD based on the analysis of clonally rearranged IGH or TCR genes and by the detection of specific translocations. While the latter are theoretically useful [51], especially for ALL with common recurring translocations including *BCR-ABL1*, *ETV6-RUNX1*, and rearrangements involving *MLL*, in practice, with the exception of *BCR-ABL1*, these are not typically used for MRD detection. In addition, some studies suggest that translocation PCR does not perform as well as either flow cytometry or antigen receptor PCR in ALL MRD detection [11].

Leukemic B lymphoblasts, like normal precursor B cells, undergo somatic recombination of the variable regions on the heavy chains of their immunoglobulin gene early in development. After insertion of random nucleotides, the variable region of each pre-B cell has a unique sequence. The clonal progeny shares the same sequence as the original cell, which molecular methods can identify with allele-specific oligonucleotide PCR primers.

Almost all B-ALLs (90%) have rearranged Ig heavy-chain genes, and approximately 60% have rearranged Ig kappa deleting elements. In addition, more than half of B-ALLs may also show clonal rearrangements of T-cell receptor genes [11]. Similarly, most T-ALL (95%) have clonal T-cell receptor gene rearrangements detectable by molecular PCR [19].

MRD detection via molecular PCR requires detection of the unique clonal gene sequence at diagnosis. Once diagnosed, the physician can follow a patient's disease throughout treatment by using PCR primers specific to the original sequence. In addition, real-time quantitative PCR (q-PCR) is able to detect the quantity of residual disease with a fluorescent reporter that increases proportionally with the amount of targeted amplicon [19].

Understandably, this process is labor-intensive and requires a high level of expertise, as well as a qualified molecular laboratory. Despite the technical hurdles, PCR is extremely sensitive and can detect MRD with a sensitivity of 10^{4-5} in >90% of B-ALL clones [44, 52]. The remaining 10% of cases undetectable with this method represent those clones that have not undergone somatic recombination [12].

Advantages and Disadvantages

When optimally performed, PCR is highly sensitive, although the exact sensitivity depends on the uniqueness of the target sequence and the quality of the specimen [19]. Moreover, largely through the efforts of the European BIOMED-2 consortium [53, 54], antigen receptor PCR is highly standardized and has been shown to be highly reproducible among performing laboratories.

TABLE 2.2 Antibodies used in the flow cytometric detection of MRD

	B-cell ALL	T-cell ALL
Consistently used	CD19,CD10,CD34,CD45,CD38	CD7,cCD3,sCD3,CD5,CD4,CD2,CD8,CD45,CD34
Common additions	CD58,CD13,CD33,CD123,CD81,CD9,CD79a,CD22[a]	Tdt,CD56[b],CD48,HLADR
May add information	CD11b,CD66c,CD24,CD304,CD73,TdT,CD15	CD99,CD38,CD13,CD33,CD117

[a]May help as a gating reagent in patients receiving anti-CD19 therapy
[b]Often used in conjunction with CD16 to help exclude NK cells

PCR also has limitations, however. High analytical sensitivity does not necessarily translate into high clinical sensitivity [12, 55, 56], and a positive PCR result may not indicate true residual disease. False-negative results are also possible, as clonal evolution may result in sequence changes which obscure MRD detection, although most protocols now require testing for at least two clonal MRD markers to prevent such false negatives. PCR methods are also labor intensive and time-consuming; the time required to synthesize and validate allele-specific primers for each patient precludes its usefulness as a tool to adjust treatment early in therapy.

Flow cytometry, on the other hand, is widely available and considerably less expensive, and results are available within hours of receipt of a specimen, making it an ideal technology to use to make rapid therapeutic decisions. In addition, flow cytometry is the only method that can be used in cases lacking the diagnostic specimen, as PCR requires knowledge of patient-specific rearrangements for allele-specific oligonucleotide primers.

One of the main challenges in flow cytometry is the lack of reproducibility due to a number of variables, including equipment, reagents, data analysis software, and reporting [57, 58]. Unlike the standardized approach to PCR methods, flow cytometry has been faulted in the past for its subjectivity in interpretation and general lack of standard approaches. While this remains a challenge, a number of efforts have been made to standardize protocols and to train laboratories operating within the context of a given protocol [11, 29, 37, 59]. BIOMED-1, a large study group composed of six different European laboratories, evaluated flow cytometry MRD protocols among different institutions. The study addressed technical issues, including reagents and instrument setup, and they achieved both high reproducibility and high concordance between laboratories [37]. However, achieving interlaboratory concordance at the level of 0.01% can still be challenging [60, 61]. The COG, which has analyzed MRD in more than 10,000 B-ALL patients using a two-tube six-color panel in two separate reference laboratories, has begun an effort to expand to include other laboratories [62]. To date, 15 laboratories have shown concordance with one of the reference laboratories using a series of a minimum of 60 split samples tested with the same panel.

Recently the EuroFlow consortium standardized a two-tube eight-color flow cytometric panel for multicenter MRD measurement using antibodies that were determined to be the most significant in discriminating between normal hematogones and ALL in multidimensional principal component analysis. With the acquisition of >4 million cells, flow cytometric detection reached a sensitivity of $<10^{-5}$, comparable to PCR. MRD results between the two methods showed a correlation of 98% [60].

Even with these efforts, the need for expert knowledge to interpret flow cytometry results remains a barrier. Much work is currently devoted to developing automated methods of data analysis. Principle component analysis-based strategies have been used successfully to classify cases of leukemia [57], but to date these methods have not been successfully employed for MRD. There have been proof of principle demonstrations of the ability to use sophisticated data analytic methods to detect MRD [63], although these have not yet been shown to be fully generalizable. Nevertheless, development of these technologies will greatly improve the utility of flow cytometric methods.

Comparison of PCR and Flow Cytometry in Clinical Studies

There has generally been good correlation between PCR and flow cytometric methods. The rate of concordance between four-color flow cytometry and PCR is reported as 70–95% [64, 65]. A multicenter study showed a concordance of 84% in detecting day 29 MRD between methods in patients with both B-ALL and T-ALL using 0.1% as a cutoff [66]. An eight-color antibody panel used in the ALL-REZ BFM study [67] was concordant with PCR results in 86.5% of samples.

Discrepancies between the methods most often arise at low-level MRD, most often with a positive PCR result and a negative flow cytometry result. This likely reflects intrinsic differences in sensitivity of the two techniques, although the specific flow cytometric protocol may also be important. In addition, nearly every study shows discrepant cases that cannot be attributed solely to differences in sensitivity. Nevertheless, on a population basis, both methods identify patient groups with differing prognosis, even if individual patients may be alternatively classified. However, due to its higher sensitivity, molecular studies are generally better at identifying a very favorable group of patients who become MRD-negative very early in response to therapy [68, 69].

Most authors agree that flow cytometry and PCR are generally concordant and may provide complementary information [49]. The choice of method for MRD detection depends on the expertise of the lab and the resources available.

Next-Generation Sequencing

New methods of DNA sequencing emerged in the late 1990s, and by 2000, high-throughput sequencing (HTS; also known as next-generation sequencing, NGS) methods were being used in a variety of research settings. Not only does NGS have the ability to sequence large quantities of DNA in a relatively short duration of time, it also has the sensitivity to quantify very small clones (1 cell in 10^{-6} cells) and to detect cells at even lower frequencies. This feature compelled researchers to begin to employ NGS methods for MRD detection, first in T-ALL and, shortly thereafter, in B-ALL [70, 71].

NGS in T-ALL

In one of the first studies of its kind, Wu et al. used HTS to assess MRD in patients with T-ALL and compared results with flow cytometry. Unique clonal TCR beta sequences and TCR gamma sequences were identified at diagnosis in 81% and 61% of patients, respectively. At day 29, they assessed MRD status in each patient using the previously defined unique clonal identifier [70]. HTS showed greater sensitivity of detection compared with flow cytometry at day 29. Those cases that were detected by HTS but not flow cytometry had clone sizes on average 10–100-fold smaller than those that were detected by both methods.

Among cases that lacked clonal TCR beta rearrangements at diagnosis, several had large clones detectable by flow cytometry at day 29 [70]. Of those cases, approximately half had an ETP immunophenotype, and approximately half had a similar phenotype except for the presence of CD5 (referred to as "near-ETP"). None of the cases with detectable clonal TCR beta rearrangements had an ETP phenotype.

NGS in B-ALL

Similar to T-ALL studies, Wu et al. used the NGS platform to sequence the IGH gene in patients with B-ALL and compared results with flow cytometry [71]. As compared with previous B-ALL NGS studies which limited testing to those patients with known IGH rearrangements [72], Wu et al. used NGS on all B-ALL patients irrespective of known IGH rearrangements and found detectable clonal rearrangements in 93% of patients in the pretreatment sample [71, 72]. In MRD-positive cases, the predominant clone in the pretreatment sample was the most frequent clone detected at day 29. As with T-ALL, there was a subset of patients with detectable MRD by NGS, but not by flow cytometry. For those cases, the average disease burden was 10–100-fold lower than the cases that were detected by both methods. Patients that lacked IGH clonal rearrangements had worse outcomes than those patients with clonal IGH, possibly because those cases represent more primitive clones [73].

NGS has advantages over both flow cytometric and conventional PCR in evaluating MRD: it is less subjective to interpretation than flow cytometry and, once the protocol is established, is less technically demanding than other molecular methods. By incorporating primers that can simultaneously amplify any possible combination of rearranged IGH or TCR loci, NGS eliminates the need for patient-specific primers. Because of this, HTS is rapid enough to use for real-time therapeutic decision-making

[70], although in current practice, it is still not as fast as flow cytometry. NGS can only detect cases with complete rearrangements, however, thereby missing a small subset of cases with no or incomplete rearrangements. As with any clone-specific PCR method, another limitation is the need for paired pretreatment and posttreatment samples. Nevertheless, NGS is a powerful method for MRD detection, as recent studies have shown that MRD detected by NGS can predict relapse and survival as accurately as flow cytometry [74] (Fig. 2.4) and conventional PCR and may ultimately replace these methods in the future [75, 76].

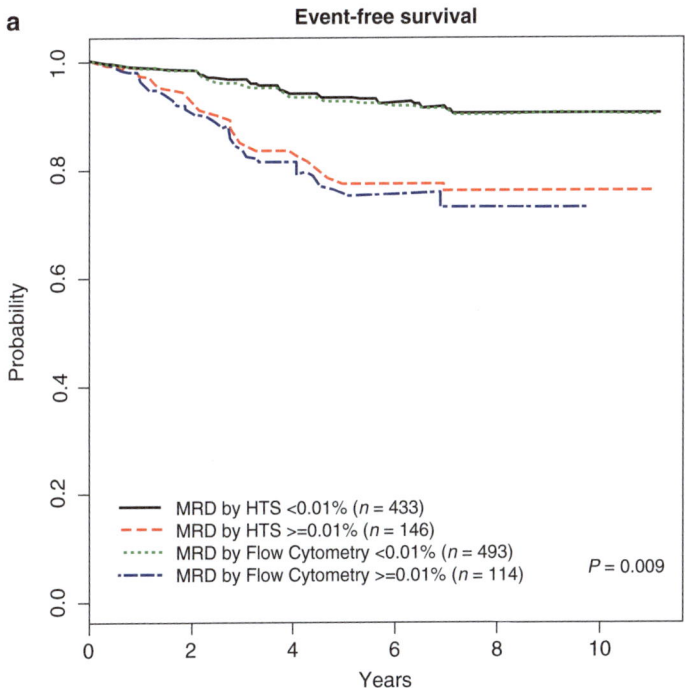

FIGURE 2.4 High-throughput sequencing (HTS) vs. flow cytometry assessment of event-free survival (EFS) and overall survival (OS)[a]. The 5-year EFS and OS for HTS and FC at a threshold of 0.01%. HTS showed similar EFS and OS to that of FC. ([a]This research was originally published in *Blood*. Wood et al. [74]. © The American Society of Hematology)

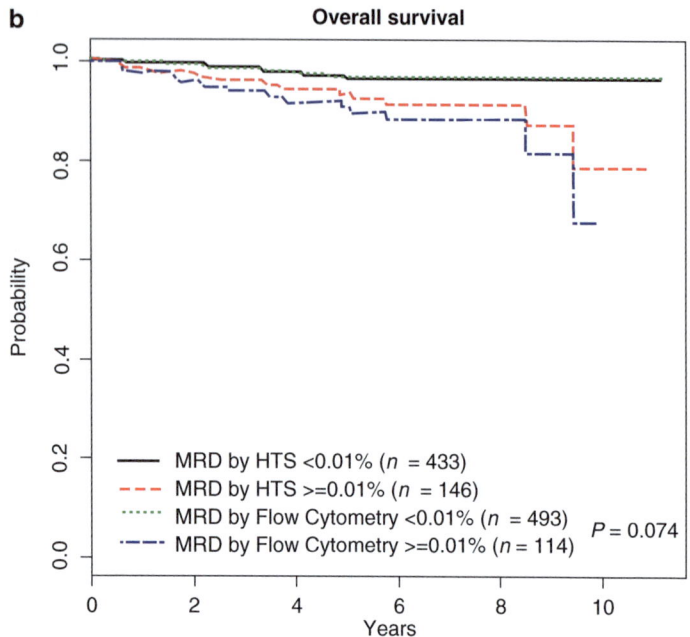

FIGURE 2.4 (continued)

Risk Stratification and the Threshold for MRD Detection

It is difficult to recommend a single level of MRD at which to intensify therapy, as the myriad of MRD studies addressing this question have used different methods of detection, with various sensitivities, at different points in time (Table 2.3). Although 0.01% is the most commonly used threshold for intervention, several lines of evidence suggest that patients with detectable MRD <0.01% early in therapy have worse outcomes than those who are truly negative. These include studies by flow cytometry [28], PCR [77], and NGS [73]. In general, these patients had statistically significant, but only marginally clinically significant, poorer outcomes; lowering the MRD threshold to capture these patients for intensification

TABLE 2.3 MRD protocols and outcomes

	Disease type	Study	Reference	Study population	MRD detection Methodology	Timing	Cutoff value	MRD-directed therapy (no. of patients)	Clinical outcome
1	Pediatric B-ALL, high-risk	AALL0232	Borowitz [29]	2473	Flow cytometry	End of induction (day 29)	0.01%	Intensified therapy to patients with MRD > 0.1% (404)	Did not improve 5-year EFS or OS. Early relapse rate similar to that seen in MRD-negative patients
2	Pediatric ALL, intermediate-risk	ALL-REZ BFM 2002	Eckert [91]	236	qPCR	End of induction (week 5)	10^{-3}	HCT (103)	Patients with MRD ≥10^{-3} who received HCT had improved probability of EFS from 18% ± 7% to 64% ± 5% and reduced CIR from 59% ± 9% to 27% ± 5%

(continued)

TABLE 2.3 MRD protocols and outcomes

Disease type	Study	Reference	MRD detection Study population	Methodology	Timing	Cutoff value	MRD-directed therapy (no. of patients)	Clinical outcome
3 Children ALL, standard-, intermediate-, and high-risk	Malaysia-Singapore ALL 2003	Yeoh [92]	556	qPCR	Day 33 and week 12	10^{-3} and 10^{-4}	Standard-risk (MRD $\leq 10^{-4}$ at day 33 and week 12) patients received deintensified subsequent therapy. Intermediate-risk (MRD $>10^{-4}$ at day 33 and $<10^{-3}$ at week 12) patients received standard therapy. High-risk (MRD $\geq 10^{-3}$ at week 12) patients received intensified therapy	6-year EFS was $93.2\% \pm 4.1\%$ in standard-risk patients, $83.6\% \pm 4.9\%$ in intermediate-risk patients, $51.8\% \pm 10\%$ in high-risk patients. 6-year OS was $95.4\% \pm 3.3\%$ in standard-risk patients, $92.1\% \pm 3.3\%$ in intermediate-risk patients, $67.7\% \pm 11\%$ in high-risk patients

| 4 | Children and young adult Ph-negative ALL, low-risk | MRC UKALL 2003 | Vora [79] | 3207 | qPCR | End of induction (day 29) and recovery from consolidation | 10^{-4} | Patients with MRD low-risk ($<10^{-4}$) received one or two delayed intensification courses (521) | No significant difference in EFS between the groups receiving one or two delayed intensification |
| 5 | Children and young adult Ph-negative ALL, standard-risk and high-risk | MRC UKALL 2003 | Vora [82] | 3207 | qPCR | End of induction (day 29) and recovery from consolidation | 10^{-4} | Patients with MRD high risk ($\geq 10^{-4}$) received standard or augmented post-remission therapy (533) | 5-year EFS was better in the augmented group than in the standard group (89.6% vs. 82.8%). OS at 5 years was numerically higher in the augmented group than in the standard group (92.9% vs. 88.9%) |

(continued)

TABLE 2.3 MRD protocols and outcomes

	Disease type	Study	Reference	Study population	MRD detection Methodology	Timing	Cutoff value	MRD-directed therapy (no. of patients)	Clinical outcome
6	Children with Ph-like B-ALL	Total Therapy XV	Roberts [93]	40	Flow cytometry and/or qPCR	End of induction remission (between day 43 and 46)	1%	HCT (6)	No significant differences in 5-year EFS (90.0% ± 4.7% vs. 88.4% ± 0.9%; P = 0.41) and OS (92.5% ± 4.2% vs. 95.1% ± 1.3%; P = 0.41) were noted between Ph-like B-ALL patients and other B-ALL subtypes
7	Children with hypodiploid ALL	Total Therapy XV and XVI	Mullighan [94]	20	Flow cytometry and/or qPCR	End of remission induction	1%	HCT (2)	The 5-year EFS was 73.6% (vs. 4-year OS 54% ± 8% in 41 hypodiploid ALL treated between 2002 and 2006)

| 8 | Pediatric ALL, low-, standard-, and high-risk | Total Therapy XV | Pui [78] | 498 | Flow cytometry and/or qPCR | Day 19 and at the end of remission induction (~day 46) and week 7 of maintenance treatment | 0.01% and 1% | Low-risk (MRD <0.01% or 0.01–0.99% at day 19 and <0.01% at day 46), standard-risk (MRD 0.01–0.99% at day 19 and 0.01–0.99% at day 46, or MRD ≥1% at day 19 and <1% at day 16), and high-risk (MRD ≥1% at day 19 and day 46) patients received risk-directed regimens. 33 received HCT | MRD ≥1% at day 19 had an unfavorable outcome: 10-year EFS 64.1% vs. 90.7% for patients with lower levels of or no detectable MRD |

(continued)

TABLE 2.3 MRD protocols and outcomes

Disease type	Study	MRD detection				MRD-directed therapy (no. of patients)	Clinical outcome
		Reference	Study population	Methodology	Timing	Cutoff value		

Disease type	Study	Reference	Study population	Methodology	Timing	Cutoff value	MRD-directed therapy (no. of patients)	Clinical outcome
9	Pediatric ALL, ALL10 standard-, intermediate-, and high-risk	Pieters [95]	778	qPCR	End of course IA (TP1) and IB (TP2)	5×10^{-4}	Standard-risk (MRD negative at TP1 and TP2) patients received reduced intensity therapy; high-risk (TP1 MRD $\geq 5 \times 10^{-4}$ or unknown and TP2 MRD $\geq 5 \times 10^{-4}$) patients received intensified therapy (some received HCT)	5-year EFS was 88.7% in ALL 10 (vs. 66.1% in ALL7, 75.4% in ALL8, and 83.3% in ALL9), and 5-year OS was 93.9% in ALL 10 (vs. 80.1% in ALL7, 85.4% in ALL8, and 88.3% in ALL9)

10	Adult Ph-negative ALL, standard-risk and high-risk	GMALL	Gokbuget [83]	1648	qPCR	Day 71 and week 16	10^{-4}	HCT (108)	Patients with MRD $\geq 10^{-4}$ who received HCT had longer probability of continuous CR after 5 years than those without HCT (66% ± 7% vs. 12% ± 5%)
11	Adult Ph-negative ALL, standard-risk and high-risk	GRAALL	Dhedin [96]	955	qPCR	6 weeks after induction initiation	10^{-3}	HCT (282)	Patients with MRD $\geq 10^{-3}$ had longer RFS. Patients with MRD $<10^{-3}$ did not benefit from HCT
12	Adult ALL	NILG-ALL 09/00	Bassan [97, 98]	280	qPCR	Week 16, week 22	10^{-4}	HCT (59)	Patients with MRD $\geq 10^{-4}$ who received HCT had improved 6-year DFS (42% vs. 18%). Posttransplant outcome was affected by post-induction MRD level

(continued)

TABLE 2.3 MRD protocols and outcomes

Disease type	Study	Reference	MRD detection Study population	Methodology	Timing	Cutoff value	MRD-directed therapy (no. of patients)	Clinical outcome
13 Adolescent and adult Ph-negative ALL, high-risk	PETHEMA ALL-AR-03	Ribera [99]	326	Flow cytometry	End of induction (weeks 5–6) and end of the third consolidation cycle (weeks 16–18)	5×10^{-4}	HCT (71)	Patients with MRD $\geq 5 \times 10^{-4}$ who received HCT had 5-year EFS and OS probability of 24% and 31%, respectively. The outcome in patients who received HCT was unfavorable, especially in patients with MRD $<5 \times 10^{-4}$

Adapted from Chen and Wood [90].© The American Society of Hematology. Reprinted by permission
ALL acute lymphoblastic leukemia, *CIR* cumulative incidence of subsequent relapse, *CR* complete remission, *DFS* disease-free survival, *EFS* event-free survival, *HCT* hematopoietic cell transplant, *MRD* minimal residual disease, *OS* overall survival, *Ph* Philadelphia chromosome, *qPCR* real-time quantitative PCR, *RFS* relapse-free survival, *TP1* time point 1, *TP2* time point 2

would result in classifying a large number of patients with good outcomes as higher risk and thus subject many more patients unnecessarily to therapy intensification. Formal cut-point analysis of both flow cytometry and NGS data recently showed that at the end of induction in B-ALL, 10^{-4} was the optimal cut point to maximally subgroup B-ALL patients by outcome [73].

By contrast, a lower threshold for MRD positivity is particularly useful to identify patients of very good risk who may benefit from reduction in therapy. Patients who are MRD negative by flow cytometry at the end of induction typically do not have a good enough outcome to be considered for such an intervention. However, patients with undetectable disease (and not merely MRD below the level of quantitation) using either q-PCR [30] or NGS [73] at this time point have excellent outcomes, with the latter identifying a cohort of NCI standard-risk patients who are essentially all cured.

However, the above comments chiefly apply to end-induction measurements, where the most data have been collected. A negative flow cytometry result earlier in therapy [23, 78] can identify patients with an excellent outcome, while at day 78, the optimal cutoff to predict poor risk is 10^{-3} rather than 10^{-4} [30, 79]. Further complicating the interpretation of MRD data is the recent demonstration that the optimal threshold for MRD cutoffs also depends upon genetic risk group [80].

Does Therapeutic Intensification Overcome the Adverse Prognostic Effect of MRD?

Once MRD was recognized as the most important prognostic factor, nearly all therapeutic studies used this parameter to assign MRD-positive patients to more intensive therapy. Therefore, there are almost no randomized data to address the question of whether therapeutic intensification can overcome the adverse prognosis of MRD. The classic randomized phase III study by Nachman et al. [81] demonstrated that intensification of therapy was effective for patients with slow early response measured by morphology, so it was logical to assume the same strategy would apply using more sensitive measures of response. Vora et al. [82] randomized intermediate-risk patients with MRD to intensification and showed that patients receiving more intensive therapy had a lower relapse rate and an improved EFS and OS. Other studies provide indirect evidence that intensification may be helpful. In prior COG trials, patients with 0.1–1% MRD at the end of induction received therapeutic intensification, while those with 0.01–0.1% MRD did not. Outcome of the former group of patients improved to match those of patients with lower levels of MRD, although in NCI high-risk patients, the improvement did not persist (Borowitz, unpublished observations, and [29]). In adult ALL, Gokbuget et al. [83] showed that bone marrow transplantation, but not conventional therapy, improved the outcome of patients with molecular failure. Finally, as noted above, patients with ETP-ALL who were given appropriately intensive therapy had an outcome equivalent to that of non-ETP patients even though they had higher levels of MRD [7].

Using MRD to Redefine Response

After induction therapy, most patients with B-ALL achieve complete remission (CR) using a standard morphologic definition. Some authors have advocated revising the definition of CR to include sensitive methods of detection instead of morphology. The Symposium on MRD assessment has proposed using terminology including "Complete MRD Response," in order to better define treatment response and to standardize methods for comparing MRD results between different treatment protocols [84]. In addition, they recommend using the terms, "MRD Persistence" and/or "MRD Reappearance," for those cases positive for MRD. The conventional definition of relapse in ALL is the reappearance of 25% blasts in the bone marrow or blood. While changing the definition of relapse to include MRD would have a significant impact on comparing clinical trials that have traditionally used the morphologic definition of relapse as a study end point, the availability of novel targeted therapies—which may work best in the minimal disease setting—has created additional need for modifying the definitions of response [85, 86]. This is also of particular importance after bone marrow transplantation, where it may be desirable to intervene therapeutically before frank relapse [87].

MRD as a Surrogate Marker of Response

Because of its early availability as an end point, it is tempting to use MRD results to assess the effectiveness of a therapy rather than waiting the many years needed to assess EFS. While a recent large meta-analysis confirmed the undeniably strong association between MRD and clinical outcomes with drugs in current use, the authors cautioned against generalized acceptance of using MRD as an end point in new drug trials. For MRD to be used as a surrogate marker, it must be shown that changes in MRD reflect changes in outcome [24]. Unfortunately, as noted above, the presence of MRD is typically used to alter therapy, so it is impossible to assess the effect of therapy on both MRD and outcome. In fact, some indirect evidence suggests that MRD may not always be a good surrogate. In a study of relapsed ALL, patients who ultimately benefited from re-induction with mitoxantrone compared with idarubicin did not show any differences in end-induction MRD levels [88]. Similarly, in a COG study of high-risk ALL, dexamethasone was shown to be superior to prednisone during induction, even though it had no effect on end-induction MRD [89]. There were flaws in both of these studies with respect to the correlation of early MRD and outcome, so this cannot be considered definitive refutation of using MRD as a surrogate. However, broad assumptions regarding MRD response to a novel agent and its effect on survival may not be appropriate. Investigators hope that the MRD response to a novel agent might translate into better outcome, but such studies still need to be done.

Summary

In summary, MRD detection has a measurable impact on the prognosis and outcomes of patients with ALL. Not only is MRD assessment a critical part of risk stratification, it also guides clinical management and treatment decisions.

The early detection of MRD-positive patients who might benefit from early intensification of therapy may be performed by flow cytometry, as it is rapid and highly sensitive. By contrast, recognizing patients with good prognosis based on lack of MRD requires more sensitive molecular methods, and NGS might be ideally suited for this purpose.

Later in therapy, it is less clear whether a high-sensitivity method of detection is beneficial, as low levels of MRD are not always associated with adverse prognosis. However, monitoring disease with a high-sensitivity method might be useful to detect early MRD conversion as a predictor of relapse, and for early intervention, although to date there are limited data to show that this strategy works.

Finally, although routine monitoring of MRD has become standard of care in the treatment of ALL, it is unclear how MRD data obtained from clinical trials that use different methods, time points, and therapies can be extrapolated to make MRD-based decisions in other circumstances. While the general assumption that MRD is a poor prognostic factor whenever it is present is probably valid, what one can or should do about such a result outside of findings from specific trials that use defined methods, time points, and treatment modalities remains unclear.

References

1. Swerdlow SH, Campo E, Pileri SA, Harris NL, Stein H, Siebert R, et al. The 2016 revision of the World Health Organization classification of lymphoid neoplasms. Blood. 2016;127(20):2375–90.
2. Coustan-Smith E, Mullighan CG, Onciu M, Behm FG, Raimondi SC, Pei D, et al. Early T-cell precursor leukaemia: a subtype of

very high-risk acute lymphoblastic leukaemia. Lancet Oncol. 2009;10(2):147–56.
3. Gaynon PS, Trigg ME, Heerema NA, Sensel MG, Sather HN, Hammond GD, et al. Children's Cancer group trials in childhood acute lymphoblastic leukemia: 1983-1995. Leukemia. 2000;14(12):2223–33.
4. Schultz KR, Pullen DJ, Sather HN, Shuster JJ, Devidas M, Borowitz MJ, et al. Risk- and response-based classification of childhood B-precursor acute lymphoblastic leukemia: a combined analysis of prognostic markers from the pediatric oncology group (POG) and Children's Cancer group (CCG). Blood. 2007;109(3):926–35.
5. Hunger SP, Loh ML, Whitlock JA, Winick NJ, Carroll WL, Devidas M, et al. Children's oncology Group's 2013 blueprint for research: acute lymphoblastic leukemia. Pediatr Blood Cancer. 2013;60(6):957–63.
6. Goldberg JM, Silverman LB, Levy DE, Dalton VK, Gelber RD, Lehmann L, et al. Childhood T-cell acute lymphoblastic leukemia: the Dana-Farber Cancer Institute acute lymphoblastic leukemia consortium experience. J Clin Oncol Off J Am Soc Clin Oncol. 2003;21(19):3616–22.
7. Wood BL, Winter SS, Dunsmore KP, Devidas M, Chen S, Asselin B, et al. T-lymphoblastic leukemia (T-ALL) shows excellent outcome, lack of significance of the early Thymic precursor (ETP) Immunophenotype, and validation of the prognostic value of end-induction minimal residual disease (MRD) in Children's oncology group (COG) study AALL0434. Blood. 2014;124(21):1.
8. Smith M, Arthur D, Camitta B, Carroll AJ, Crist W, Gaynon P, Gelber R, Heerema N, Korn EL, Link M, Murphy S, Pui CH, Pullen J, Reamon G, Sallan SE, Sather H, Shuster J, Simon R, Trigg M, Tubergen D, Ucken F, Ungerleider R. "Uniform approach to risk classifciation and treatment assignment for children with acute lymphoblastic leukemia." J Clin Oncol. 1996;14(1):18–24.
9. Pullen J, Shuster JJ, Link M, Borowitz M, Amylon M, Carroll AJ, et al. Significance of commonly used prognostic factors differs for children with T cell acute lymphocytic leukemia (ALL), as compared to those with B-precursor ALL. A pediatric oncology group (POG) study. Leukemia. 1999;13(11):1696–707.
10. Coustan-Smith E, Sancho J, Hancock ML, Razzouk BI, Ribeiro RC, Rivera GK, et al. Use of peripheral blood instead of bone marrow to monitor residual disease in children with acute lymphoblastic leukemia. Blood. 2002;100(7):2399–402.

11. Gaipa G, Basso G, Biondi A, Campana D. Detection of minimal residual disease in pediatric acute lymphoblastic leukemia. Cytometry B Clin Cytom. 2013;84(6):359–69.
12. Campana D, Pui CH. Detection of minimal residual disease in acute leukemia: methodologic advances and clinical significance. Blood. 1995;85(6):1416–34.
13. Cave H, van der Werff ten Bosch J, Suciu S, Guidal C, Waterkeyn C, Otten J, et al. Clinical significance of minimal residual disease in childhood acute lymphoblastic leukemia. European Organization for Research and Treatment of Cancer--childhood leukemia cooperative group. N Engl J Med. 1998;339(9):591–8.
14. Coustan-Smith E, Behm FG, Sanchez J, Boyett JM, Hancock ML, Raimondi SC, et al. Immunological detection of minimal residual disease in children with acute lymphoblastic leukaemia. Lancet. 1998;351(9102):550–4.
15. Coustan-Smith E, Sancho J, Hancock ML, Boyett JM, Behm FG, Raimondi SC, et al. Clinical importance of minimal residual disease in childhood acute lymphoblastic leukemia. Blood. 2000;96(8):2691–6.
16. Farahat N, Morilla A, Owusu-Ankomah K, Morilla R, Pinkerton CR, Treleaven JG, et al. Detection of minimal residual disease in B-lineage acute lymphoblastic leukaemia by quantitative flow cytometry. Br J Haematol. 1998;101(1):158–64.
17. Farahat N, Lens D, Zomas A, Morilla R, Matutes E, Catovsky D. Quantitative flow cytometry can distinguish between normal and leukaemic B-cell precursors. Br J Haematol. 1995;91(3):640–6.
18. Campana D, Neale GA, Coustan-Smith E, Pui CH. Detection of minimal residual disease in acute lymphoblastic leukaemia: the St Jude experience. Leukemia. 2001;15(2):278–9.
19. Campana D. Determination of minimal residual disease in leukaemia patients. Br J Haematol. 2003;121(6):823–38.
20. Ciudad J, San Miguel JF, Lopez-Berges MC, Vidriales B, Valverde B, Ocqueteau M, et al. Prognostic value of immunophenotypic detection of minimal residual disease in acute lymphoblastic leukemia. J Clin Oncol Off J Am Soc Clin Oncol. 1998;16(12):3774–81.
21. Campana D. Applications of cytometry to study acute leukemia: in vitro determination of drug sensitivity and detection of minimal residual disease. Cytometry. 1994;18(2):68–74.
22. Brisco MJ, Condon J, Hughes E, Neoh SH, Sykes PJ, Seshadri R, et al. Outcome prediction in childhood acute lymphoblastic

leukaemia by molecular quantification of residual disease at the end of induction. Lancet. 1994;343(8891):196–200.
23. Basso G, Veltroni M, Valsecchi MG, Dworzak MN, Ratei R, Silvestri D, et al. Risk of relapse of childhood acute lymphoblastic leukemia is predicted by flow cytometric measurement of residual disease on day 15 bone marrow. J Clin Oncol Off J Am Soc Clin Oncol. 2009;27(31):5168–74.
24. Berry DA, Zhou S, Higley H, Mukundan L, Fu S, Reaman GH, et al. Association of Minimal Residual Disease with Clinical Outcome in pediatric and adult acute lymphoblastic leukemia: a meta-analysis. JAMA Oncol. 2017;3(7):e170580.
25. Hunger SP, Mullighan CG. Acute lymphoblastic leukemia in children. N Engl J Med. 2015;373(16):1541–52.
26. van Dongen JJ, Seriu T, Panzer-Grumayer ER, Biondi A, Pongers-Willemse MJ, Corral L, et al. Prognostic value of minimal residual disease in acute lymphoblastic leukaemia in childhood. Lancet. 1998;352(9142):1731–8.
27. Biondi A, Valsecchi MG, Seriu T, D'Aniello E, Willemse MJ, Fasching K, et al. Molecular detection of minimal residual disease is a strong predictive factor of relapse in childhood B-lineage acute lymphoblastic leukemia with medium risk features. A case control study of the international BFM study group. Leukemia. 2000;14(11):1939–43.
28. Borowitz MJ, Devidas M, Hunger SP, Bowman WP, Carroll AJ, Carroll WL, et al. Clinical significance of minimal residual disease in childhood acute lymphoblastic leukemia and its relationship to other prognostic factors: a Children's oncology group study. Blood. 2008;111(12):5477–85.
29. Borowitz MJ, Wood BL, Devidas M, Loh ML, Raetz EA, Salzer WL, et al. Prognostic significance of minimal residual disease in high risk B-ALL: a report from Children's oncology group study AALL0232. Blood. 2015;126(8):964–71.
30. Conter V, Bartram CR, Valsecchi MG, Schrauder A, Panzer-Grumayer R, Moricke A, et al. Molecular response to treatment redefines all prognostic factors in children and adolescents with B-cell precursor acute lymphoblastic leukemia: results in 3184 patients of the AIEOP-BFM ALL 2000 study. Blood. 2010;115(16):3206–14.
31. Conter V, Arico M, Basso G, Biondi A, Barisone E, Messina C, et al. Long-term results of the Italian Association of Pediatric Hematology and Oncology (AIEOP) studies 82, 87, 88, 91 and

95 for childhood acute lymphoblastic leukemia. Leukemia. 2010;24(2):255–64.
32. Schrappe M, Valsecchi MG, Bartram CR, Schrauder A, Panzer-Grumayer R, Moricke A, et al. Late MRD response determines relapse risk overall and in subsets of childhood T-cell ALL: results of the AIEOP-BFM-ALL 2000 study. Blood. 2011;118(8):2077–84.
33. Mancini M, Cedrone M, Diverio D, Emanuel B, Stul M, Vranckx H, et al. Use of dual-color interphase FISH for the detection of inv(16) in acute myeloid leukemia at diagnosis, relapse and during follow-up: a study of 23 patients. Leukemia. 2000;14(3):364–8.
34. Bielorai B, Golan H, Trakhtenbrot L, Reichart M, Toren A, Daniely M, et al. Combined analysis of morphology and fluorescence in situ hybridization in follow-up of minimal residual disease in a child with Philadelphia-positive acute lymphoblastic leukemia. Cancer Genet Cytogenet. 2002;138(1):64–8.
35. Weir EG, Cowan K, LeBeau P, Borowitz MJ. A limited antibody panel can distinguish B-precursor acute lymphoblastic leukemia from normal B precursors with four color flow cytometry: implications for residual disease detection. Leukemia. 1999;13(4):558–67.
36. Roshal M, Fromm JR, Winter S, Dunsmore K, Wood BL. Immaturity associated antigens are lost during induction for T cell lymphoblastic leukemia: implications for minimal residual disease detection. Cytometry B Clin Cytom. 2010;78((3):139–46.
37. Lucio P, Parreira A, van den Beemd MW, van Lochem EG, van Wering ER, Baars E, et al. Flow cytometric analysis of normal B cell differentiation: a frame of reference for the detection of minimal residual disease in precursor-B-ALL. Leukemia. 1999;13(3):419–27.
38. Dworzak MN, Fritsch G, Panzer-Grumayer ER, Mann G, Gadner H. Detection of residual disease in pediatric B-cell precursor acute lymphoblastic leukemia by comparative phenotype mapping: method and significance. Leuk Lymphoma. 2000;38(3–4):295–308.
39. Borowitz MJ, Pullen DJ, Winick N, Martin PL, Bowman WP, Camitta B. Comparison of diagnostic and relapse flow cytometry phenotypes in childhood acute lymphoblastic leukemia: implications for residual disease detection: a report from the children's oncology group. Cytometry B Clin Cytom. 2005;68((1):18–24.
40. Gaipa G, Basso G, Maglia O, Leoni V, Faini A, Cazzaniga G, et al. Drug-induced immunophenotypic modulation in child-

hood ALL: implications for minimal residual disease detection. Leukemia. 2005;19(1):49–56.
41. Dworzak MN, Schumich A, Printz D, Potschger U, Husak Z, Attarbaschi A, et al. CD20 up-regulation in pediatric B-cell precursor acute lymphoblastic leukemia during induction treatment: setting the stage for anti-CD20 directed immunotherapy. Blood. 2008;112(10):3982–8.
42. Wood B. Multicolor immunophenotyping: human immune system hematopoiesis. Methods Cell Biol. 2004;75:559–76.
43. Pui CH, Behm FG, Crist WM. Clinical and biologic relevance of immunologic marker studies in childhood acute lymphoblastic leukemia. Blood. 1993;82(2):343–62.
44. van Dongen JJ, Breit TM, Adriaansen HJ, Beishuizen A, Hooijkaas H. Detection of minimal residual disease in acute leukemia by immunological marker analysis and polymerase chain reaction. Leukemia. 1992;6(Suppl 1):47–59.
45. Campana D, Coustan-Smith E, Behm FG. The definition of remission in acute leukemia with immunologic techniques. Bone Marrow Transplant. 1991;8(6):429–37.
46. Bjorklund E, Mazur J, Soderhall S, Porwit-MacDonald A. Flow cytometric follow-up of minimal residual disease in bone marrow gives prognostic information in children with acute lymphoblastic leukemia. Leukemia. 2003;17(1):138–48.
47. Shaver AC, Greig BW, Mosse CA, Seegmiller AC. B-ALL minimal residual disease flow cytometry: an application of a novel method for optimization of a single-tube model. Am J Clin Pathol. 2015;143(5):716–24.
48. Borowitz MJ, Pullen DJ, Shuster JJ, Viswanatha D, Montgomery K, Willman CL, et al. Minimal residual disease detection in childhood precursor-B-cell acute lymphoblastic leukemia: relation to other risk factors. A Children's oncology group study. Leukemia. 2003;17(8):1566–72.
49. Gaipa G, Cazzaniga G, Valsecchi MG, Panzer-Grumayer R, Buldini B, Silvestri D, et al. Time point-dependent concordance of flow cytometry and real-time quantitative polymerase chain reaction for minimal residual disease detection in childhood acute lymphoblastic leukemia. Haematologica. 2012;97(10):1582–93.
50. Perfetto SP, Ambrozak D, Nguyen R, Chattopadhyay P, Roederer M. Quality assurance for polychromatic flow cytometry. Nat Protoc. 2006;1(3):1522–30.
51. Roberts KG, Reshmi SC, Harvey RC, Chen IM, Patel K, Stonerock E, Jenkins H, Dai Y, Valentine M, Gu Z, Zhao Y, Zhang J, Payne-Turner

D, Devidas M, Heerema NA, Carroll AJ, Raetz EA, Borowitz MJ, Wood BL, Mattano LA Jr, Maloney KW, Carroll WL, Loh ML, Willman CL, Gastier-Foster JM, Mullighan CG, Hunger SP. "Genomic and outcome analyses of PH-like ALL in NCI standard-risk patients: a report from the Children's Oncology Group." Blood. 2018;132(8):815–24.
52. Campana D, Yokota S, Coustan-Smith E, Hansen-Hagge TE, Janossy G, Bartram CR. The detection of residual acute lymphoblastic leukemia cells with immunologic methods and polymerase chain reaction: a comparative study. Leukemia. 1990;4(9):609–14.
53. van der Velden VH, Panzer-Grumayer ER, Cazzaniga G, Flohr T, Sutton R, Schrauder A, et al. Optimization of PCR-based minimal residual disease diagnostics for childhood acute lymphoblastic leukemia in a multi-center setting. Leukemia. 2007;21(4):706–13.
54. van der Velden VH, van Dongen JJ. MRD detection in acute lymphoblastic leukemia patients using Ig/TCR gene rearrangements as targets for real-time quantitative PCR. Methods Mol Biol (Clifton, NJ). 2009;538:115–50.
55. Beishuizen A, Verhoeven MA, van Wering ER, Hahlen K, Hooijkaas H, van Dongen JJ. Analysis of Ig and T-cell receptor genes in 40 childhood acute lymphoblastic leukemias at diagnosis and subsequent relapse: implications for the detection of minimal residual disease by polymerase chain reaction analysis. Blood. 1994;83(8):2238–47.
56. Yokota S, Hansen-Hagge TE, Ludwig WD, Reiter A, Raghavachar A, Kleihauer E, et al. Use of polymerase chain reactions to monitor minimal residual disease in acute lymphoblastic leukemia patients. Blood. 1991;77(2):331–9.
57. van Dongen JJ, Lhermitte L, Bottcher S, Almeida J, van der Velden VH, Flores-Montero J, et al. EuroFlow antibody panels for standardized n-dimensional flow cytometric immunophenotyping of normal, reactive and malignant leukocytes. Leukemia. 2012;26(9):1908–75.
58. Greig B, Oldaker T, Warzynski M, Wood B. 2006 Bethesda international consensus recommendations on the immunophenotypic analysis of hematolymphoid neoplasia by flow cytometry: recommendations for training and education to perform clinical flow cytometry. Cytometry B Clin Cytom. 2007;72(Suppl 1):S23–33.
59. Irving J, Jesson J, Virgo P, Case M, Minto L, Eyre L, et al. Establishment and validation of a standard protocol for the

detection of minimal residual disease in B lineage childhood acute lymphoblastic leukemia by flow cytometry in a multicenter setting. Haematologica. 2009;94(6):870–4.
60. Theunissen P, Mejstrikova E, Sedek L, van der Sluijs-Gelling AJ, Gaipa G, Bartels M, et al. Standardized flow cytometry for highly sensitive MRD measurements in B-cell acute lymphoblastic leukemia. Blood. 2017;129(3):347–57.
61. Dworzak MN, Froschl G, Printz D, Mann G, Potschger U, Muhlegger N, et al. Prognostic significance and modalities of flow cytometric minimal residual disease detection in childhood acute lymphoblastic leukemia. Blood. 2002;99(6):1952–8.
62. Keeney M, Wood BL, Hedley BD, DiGiuseppe JA, Stetler-Stevenson M, Paietta E, et al. A QA program for MRD testing demonstrates that systematic education can reduce discordance among experienced interpreters. Cytometry B Clin Cytom. 2017;94:239.
63. DiGiuseppe JA, Tadmor MD, Pe'er D. Detection of minimal residual disease in B lymphoblastic leukemia using viSNE. Cytometry B Clin Cytom. 2015;88(5):294–304.
64. Neale GA, Coustan-Smith E, Pan Q, Chen X, Gruhn B, Stow P, et al. Tandem application of flow cytometry and polymerase chain reaction for comprehensive detection of minimal residual disease in childhood acute lymphoblastic leukemia. Leukemia. 1999;13(8):1221–6.
65. Munoz L, Lopez O, Martino R, Brunet S, Bellido M, Rubiol E, et al. Combined use of reverse transcriptase polymerase chain reaction and flow cytometry to study minimal residual disease in Philadelphia positive acute lymphoblastic leukemia. Haematologica. 2000;85(7):704–10.
66. Thorn I, Forestier E, Botling J, Thuresson B, Wasslavik C, Bjorklund E, et al. Minimal residual disease assessment in childhood acute lymphoblastic leukaemia: a Swedish multi-Centre study comparing real-time polymerase chain reaction and multicolour flow cytometry. Br J Haematol. 2011;152(6):743–53.
67. Karawajew L, Dworzak M, Ratei R, Rhein P, Gaipa G, Buldini B, et al. Minimal residual disease analysis by eight-color flow cytometry in relapsed childhood acute lymphoblastic leukemia. Haematologica. 2015;100(7):935–44.
68. Panzer-Grumayer ER, Schneider M, Panzer S, Fasching K, Gadner H. Rapid molecular response during early induction chemotherapy predicts a good outcome in childhood acute lymphoblastic leukemia. Blood. 2000;95(3):790–4.

69. Sutton R, Venn NC, Tolisano J, Bahar AY, Giles JE, Ashton LJ, et al. Clinical significance of minimal residual disease at day 15 and at the end of therapy in childhood acute lymphoblastic leukaemia. Br J Haematol. 2009;146(3):292–9.
70. Wu D, Sherwood A, Fromm JR, Winter SS, Dunsmore KP, Loh ML, et al. High-throughput sequencing detects minimal residual disease in acute T lymphoblastic leukemia. Sci Transl Med. 2012;4(134):134ra63.
71. Wu D, Emerson RO, Sherwood A, Loh ML, Angiolillo A, Howie B, et al. Detection of minimal residual disease in B lymphoblastic leukemia by high-throughput sequencing of IGH. Clin Cancer Res Off Am Assoc Cancer Res. 2014;20(17):4540–8.
72. Faham M, Zheng J, Moorhead M, Carlton VE, Stow P, Coustan-Smith E, et al. Deep-sequencing approach for minimal residual disease detection in acute lymphoblastic leukemia. Blood. 2012;120(26):5173–80.
73. Wood BL, Wu D, Kirsch IM, Crossley B, Williamson D, Gawad C, et al. Residual disease monitoring by high throughput sequencing provides risk stratification in childhood B-ALL and identifies a novel subset of patients having poor outcome. Blood. 2016;128(22):1086.
74. Wood B, Wu D, Crossley B, Dai Y, Williamson D, Gawad C, et al. Measurable residual disease detection by high throughput sequencing improves risk stratification for pediatric B-ALL. Blood. 2017;131:1350.
75. Pulsipher MA, Carlson C, Langholz B, Wall DA, Schultz KR, Bunin N, et al. IgH-V(D)J NGS-MRD measurement pre- and early post-allotransplant defines very low- and very high-risk ALL patients. Blood. 2015;125(22):3501–8.
76. Kotrova M, Muzikova K, Mejstrikova E, Novakova M, Bakardjieva-Mihaylova V, Fiser K, et al. The predictive strength of next-generation sequencing MRD detection for relapse compared with current methods in childhood ALL. Blood. 2015;126(8):1045–7.
77. Paganin M, Fabbri G, Conter V, Barisone E, Polato K, Cazzaniga G, et al. Postinduction minimal residual disease monitoring by polymerase chain reaction in children with acute lymphoblastic leukemia. J Clin Oncol Off J Am Soc Clin Oncol. 2014;32(31):3553–8.
78. Pui CH, Pei D, Coustan-Smith E, Jeha S, Cheng C, Bowman WP, et al. Clinical utility of sequential minimal residual disease measurements in the context of risk-based therapy in childhood

acute lymphoblastic leukaemia: a prospective study. Lancet Oncol. 2015;16(4):465–74.
79. Vora A, Goulden N, Wade R, Mitchell C, Hancock J, Hough R, et al. Treatment reduction for children and young adults with low-risk acute lymphoblastic leukaemia defined by minimal residual disease (UKALL 2003): a randomised controlled trial. Lancet Oncol. 2013;14(3):199–209.
80. O'Connor D, Enshaei A, Bartram J, Hancock J, Harrison CJ, Hough R, et al. Genotype-specific minimal residual disease interpretation improves stratification in pediatric acute lymphoblastic leukemia. J Clin Oncol Off J Am Soc Clin Oncol. 2018;36(1):34–43.
81. Nachman JB, Sather HN, Sensel MG, Trigg ME, Cherlow JM, Lukens JN, et al. Augmented post-induction therapy for children with high-risk acute lymphoblastic leukemia and a slow response to initial therapy. N Engl J Med. 1998;338(23):1663–71.
82. Vora A, Goulden N, Mitchell C, Hancock J, Hough R, Rowntree C, et al. Augmented post-remission therapy for a minimal residual disease-defined high-risk subgroup of children and young people with clinical standard-risk and intermediate-risk acute lymphoblastic leukaemia (UKALL 2003): a randomised controlled trial. Lancet Oncol. 2014;15(8):809–18.
83. Gokbuget N, Kneba M, Raff T, Trautmann H, Bartram CR, Arnold R, et al. Adult patients with acute lymphoblastic leukemia and molecular failure display a poor prognosis and are candidates for stem cell transplantation and targeted therapies. Blood. 2012;120(9):1868–76.
84. Bruggemann M, Schrauder A, Raff T, Pfeifer H, Dworzak M, Ottmann OG, et al. Standardized MRD quantification in European ALL trials: proceedings of the second international symposium on MRD assessment in Kiel, Germany, 18-20 September 2008. Leukemia. 2010;24(3):521–35.
85. Ronson A, Tvito A, Rowe JM. Treatment of Philadelphia chromosome-positive acute lymphocytic leukemia. Curr Treat Options in Oncol. 2017;18(3):20.
86. Naddafi F, Davami F. Anti-CD19 monoclonal antibodies: a new approach to lymphoma therapy. Int J Mol Cell Med. 2015;4(3):143–51.
87. Kroger N, Bacher U, Bader P, Bottcher S, Borowitz MJ, Dreger P, et al. NCI first international workshop on the biology, prevention, and treatment of relapse after allogeneic hematopoietic stem cell transplantation: report from the committee

on disease-specific methods and strategies for monitoring relapse following allogeneic stem cell transplantation. Part II: chronic leukemias, myeloproliferative neoplasms, and lymphoid malignancies. Biol Blood Marrow Transplant. J Am Soc Blood Marrow Transplant. 2010;16(10):1325–46.
88. Parker C, Waters R, Leighton C, Hancock J, Sutton R, Moorman AV, et al. Effect of mitoxantrone on outcome of children with first relapse of acute lymphoblastic leukaemia (ALL R3): an open-label randomised trial. Lancet. 2010;376(9757):2009–17.
89. Larsen EC, Devidas M, Chen S, Salzer WL, Raetz EA, Loh ML, et al. Dexamethasone and high-dose methotrexate improve outcome for children and young adults with high-risk B-acute lymphoblastic leukemia: a report from Children's oncology group study AALL0232. J Clin Oncol Off J Am Soc Clin Oncol. 2016;34(20):2380–8.
90. Chen X, Wood BL. Monitoring minimal residual disease in acute leukemia: technical challenges and interpretive complexities. Blood Rev. 2017;31(2):63–75.
91. Eckert C, Henze G, Seeger K, Hagedorn N, Mann G, Panzer-Grumayer R, Peters C, Klingebiel T, Borkhardt A, Schrappe M, Schrauder A, Escherich G, Sramkova L, Niggli F, Hitzler J, von Stackelberg A. Use of allogeneic hematopoietic stem-cell transplantation based on minimal residual disease response improves outcomes for children with relapsed acute lymphoblastic leukemia in the intermediate-risk group. J Clin Oncol. 2013;31(21):2736–42.
92. Yeoh AE, Ariffin H, Chai EL, Kwok CS, Chan YH, Ponnudurai K, Campana D, Tan PL, Chan MY, Kham SK, Chong LA, Tan AM, Lin HP, Quah TC. Minimal residual disease-guided treatment deintensification for children with acute lymphoblastic leukemia; results from the Malaysia-Singapore acute lymphoblastic leukemia 2003 study. J Clin Oncol. 2012;30(19):2384–92.
93. Roberts KG, Pei D, Campana D, Payne-Turner D, Li Y, Cheng C, Sandlund JT, Jeha S, Easton J, Becksfort J, Zhang J, Coustan-Smith E, Raimondi SC, Leung WH, Relling MV, Evans WE, Downing JR, Mullighan CG, Pui CH. Outcomes of children with BCR-ABL1-like acute lymphoblastic leukemia treated with risk-directed therapy based on the levels of minimal residual disease. J Clin Oncol. 2014;32(27):3012–20.
94. Mullighan CG, Jeha S, Pei D, Payne-Turner D, Coustan-Smith E, Roberts KG, Waanders E, Choi JK, Ma X, Raimondi SC,

Fan Y, Yang W, Song G, Yang JJ, Inaba H, Downing JR, Leung WH, Bowman WP, Relling MV, Evans WE, Zhang J, Campana D, Pui CH. Outcome of children with hypodiploid ALL treated with risk-directed therapy based on MRD levels. Blood. 2015;126(26):2896–9.

95. Pieters R, de Groot-Kruseman H, Van der Velden V, Fiocco M, van den Berg H, de Bont E, Egeler RM, Hoogerbrugge P, Kaspers G, Van der Schoot E, De Haas V, Van Dongen J. Successful therapy reduction and intensification for childhood acute lymphoblastic leukemia based on minimal residual disease monitoring: study ALL 10 from the Dutch childhood oncology group. J Clin Oncol. 2016;34(22):2591–601.

96. Dhédin N, Huynh A, Maury S, Tabrizi R, Beldjord K, Asnafi V, Thomas X, Chevallier P, Nguyen S, Coiteux V, Bourhis JH, Hichri Y, Escoffre-Barbe M, Reman O, Graux C, Chalandon Y, Blaise D, Schanz U, Lhéritier V, Cahn JY, Dombret H, Ifrah N, GRAALL group. Role of allogeneic stem cell transplantation in adult patients with PH-negative acute lymphoblastic leukemia. Blood. 2015;125(16):2486–96.

97. Bassan R, Spinelli O, Oldani E, Intermesoli T, Tosi M, Peruta B, Rossi G, Borlenghi E, Pogliani EM, Terruzzi E, Fabris P, Cassibba V, Lambertenghi-Deliliers G, Cortelezzi A, Bosi A, Gianfaldoni G, Ciceri F, Bernardi M, Gallamini A, Mattei D, Di Bona E, Romani C, Scattolin AM, Barbui T, Rambaldi A. Improved risk classification for risk-specific therapy based on the molecular study of minimal residual disease (MRD) in adult acute lymphoblastic leukemia (ALL). Blood. 2009;113(18):4153–62.

98. Bassan R, Spinelli O, Oldani E, Intermesoli T, Tosi M, Peruta B, Borlenghi E, Pogliani EM, Di Bona E, Cassibba V, Scattolin AM, Romani C, Ciceri F, Cortelezzi A, Gianfaldoni G, Mattei D, Audisio E, Rambaldi A. Different molecular levels of post-induction minimal residual disease may predict hematopoietic stem cell transplantation outcome in adult Philadelphia-negative acute lymphoblastic leukemia. Blood Cancer J. 2014;11(4):e225.

99. Ribera JM, Oriol A, Morgades M, Montesinos P, Sarrà J, González-Campos J, Brunet S, Tormo M, Fernández-Abellán P, Guàrdia R, Bernal MT, Esteve J, Barba P, Moreno MJ, Bermúdez A, Cladera A, Escoda L, García-Boyero R, Del Potro E, Bergua J, Amigo ML, Grande C, Rabuñal MJ, Hernández-Rivas JM,

Feliu E. Treament of high-risk Philadelphia chromosome-negative acute lymphoblastic leukemia in adolescents and adults according to early cytologic response and minimal resiudal disease after consolidation assessed by flow cytometry: final results of the PETHEMA ALL-AR-03 trial. J Clin Onocl. 2014;32(15):1595–604.

Chapter 3
Molecular Diagnostics for Minimal Residual Disease Analysis in Hematopoietic Malignancies

Barbara K. Zehentner

Introduction

Several studies have shown that quantitative detection of minimal residual disease, or more accurately termed measurable residual disease (MRD), in lymphoid as well as myeloid malignancies can predict clinical outcome [1–10].

Monitoring treatment response by tumor load quantification is crucial to assess risk of relapse and for determining those patients who may benefit from therapy reduction, intensification, reduction of immunosuppression for graft-versus-leukemia effect post stem cell transplant, or adoptive T-cell therapy [11]. MRD negativity implies that no residual disease is detected with high certainty using a technique that can reliably measure $\leq 10^{-4}$. Two specific and sensitive testing modalities currently meet this specification, namely, multiparameter flow cytometry (MFC) as well as molecular protocols. The latter are often considered as a

---

B. K. Zehentner
Hematologics Inc., Seattle, WA, USA
e-mail: barbara@hematologics.com

method of choice if tumor-specific molecular targets can be identified, since detection limits can often reach 10^{-5} or even 10^{-6}.

RQ-PCR

Real-time quantitative RT-PCR (RQ-PCR) presents itself as a sensitive as well as specific tool to monitor measurable or minimal residual disease (MRD) in leukemic patients. Most commonly, the amplification of fusion gene transcripts is targeted by this technology. RNA products resulting from chromosomal translocations unique to leukemic cells are reverse transcribed into cDNA and subsequently amplified using specific primer and probe sets (Fig. 3.1). Leukemia-associated fusion genes are directly linked to leukemogenesis and represent very good and stable disease-specific markers throughout treatment [12]. Assays routinely achieve sensitivity levels of 1 in 10^5 (0.001%: 1 malignant cell among 100,000 normal cells). Furthermore, if a diagnostic specimen was evaluated for the presence of a fusion transcript using the identical assay platform, high specificity can be assumed. Since RNA is highly susceptible to degradation, specimens have to be processed within 24–72 h after collection. Thanks to large standardization efforts and consensus guidelines (e.g., BIOMED-1, EAC, International Standard for Bcr-Abl), several assay designs are universally available for uniform patient groups. However, assay validations as well as monitoring algorithms still have to be carefully designed and overseen in each individual laboratory, in order to prevent false-negative or false-positive findings and to ensure accurate quantification.

BCR-ABL1

Quantitative monitoring of *BCR-ABL1* transcripts is the poster child of a successful molecular diagnostic assay in the modern era of oncology. Not only can the test be used for the detection of t(9;22) during the diagnostic workup for chronic myeloid leukemia (CML), acute lymphoid leukemia

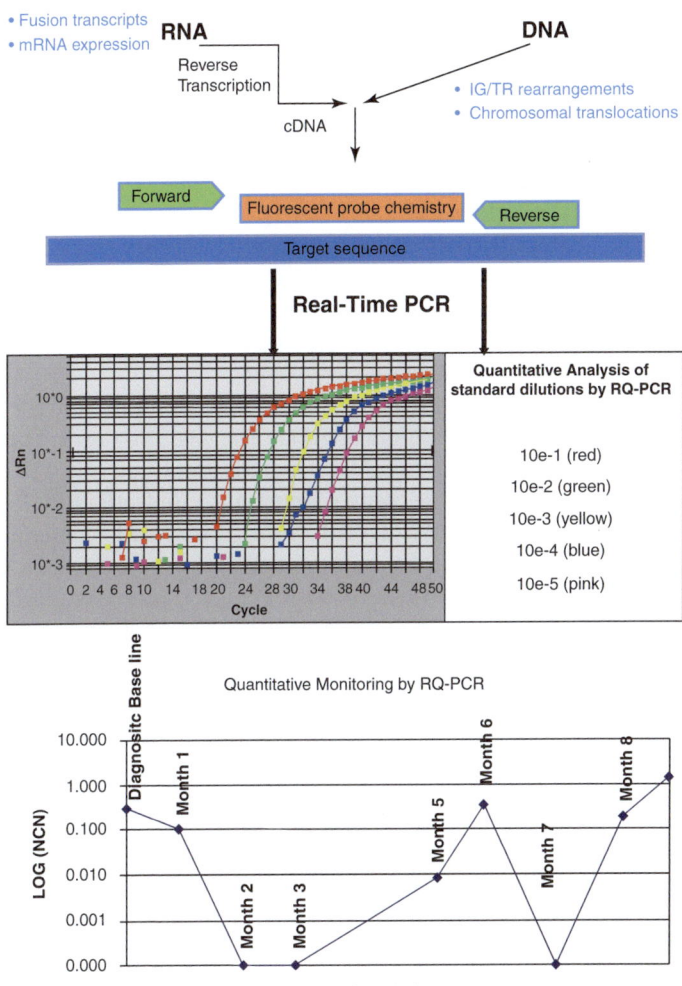

FIGURE 3.1 Real-time quantitative PCR (RQ-PCR)

(ALL), and acute myeloid leukemia (AML) but also to monitor treatment response and residual disease. Quantitative *BCR-ABL1* monitoring is currently being used to assess if optimal response is achieved in a timely manner. In CML, outcome predictions as well as risk of progression to accelerated phase and blast crisis have been associated with molecular response kinetics [13]. Standardization and optimization efforts of *BCR-ABL1* RQ-PCR testing are briefly reviewed in this chapter, since they represent hallmarks for all subsequent RQ-PCR platforms. Commercially available BCR-ABL1 test kits may only detect M-bcr (major breakpoint cluster region) b2a2 (e13a2) and b3a2 (e14a2) transcripts encoding the 210 kDA (p210) chimeric tyrosine kinase protein. However, many reference laboratories also offer simultanous or separate BCR-ABL1 testing for the m-bcr (minor breakpoint cluster region) e1-a2 transcript encoding the 190 kDA (p190) protein or even more rare BCR-ABL1 breakpoints.

BCR-ABL1 testing itself has gone through multiple iterations of standardization throughout the last 15 years. The Europe Against Cancer (EAC) program identified the ABL gene as the most reliable control gene transcript for RQ-PCR-based diagnosis and MRD detection in leukemic patients [14]. The achievement of a major molecular response (MMR) with *BCR-ABL1* values $\leq 0.10\%$ on the international reporting scale (IS) has been defined as a clinical goal. In recent years, even deeper molecular response rates have been targeted, with the development of more sensitive monitoring assays. A deep molecular response is reported if *BCR-ABL1* values reach $\leq 0.01\%$ IS. Additional cutoff values of molecular response 4 (MR4) $\leq 0.01\%$ IS, MR 4.5 $\leq 0.0032\%$ IS, and MR5 $< 0.001\%$ IS have been recently defined [15, 16]. Consequently, major molecular response (MMR) would correspond to MR3, with a 3-log reduction from a standardized baseline. Standard quantitative PCR platforms should routinely achieve MR4; however, the quality and age of the sample as well as the isolated RNA specimen have to be taken into consideration. Reaching a *BCR-ABL1* level of $<1\%$ IS, which is the equivalent to CCyR (complete cytogenetic response), by 3 months has strongly been associated with high rates of deep molecular response in CML [17]. Furthermore, reaching MMR by 12 months has been correlated with optimal response. However, even with harmonized procedures using the international standard (IS) scale, inherent variability of molecular assays has to be taken into account [13]. Despite standardization of quantification strategies, the variability around clinically relevant cutoff values may still vary greatly from laboratory to laboratory [13]. Using the identical laboratory as well as standardized test methods for individual patient monitoring can provide some consistency. The International Scale (IS) standards based on the International Randomized Study of Interferon and STI571 (IRIS) are now commercially available and uniformly applied for *BCR-ABL1* testing. However, the use of patient-specific standards and calculations was originally defined by the Europe Against Cancer (EAC) consortium [14, 18]. Despite newly implemented international standardizations, the continued use of patient-specific baseline specimens, as well as routine side-by-side testing of patient-specific monitoring specimens, can provide great value as quantification controls. This approach, in addition to the use of IS standards, can normalize for intrinsic assay variations, allowing more accurate determination of patient-specific response rates and trends. Furthermore, European LeukemiaNet (ELN) consensus guidelines for MRD assessment by PCR recommend testing to be performed in triplicates [19]. With costly commercial platforms being established in numerous laboratories, duplicate or even single-tube testing has been adopted in routine clinical testing. However, this newly implemented practice effectively reduces accuracy of quantitative findings as well as increases the likelihood of false-positive or false-negative results. In addition, the ELN consensus document recommends the side-by-side measurement of two patient-specific samples after conversion of MRD from negative to positive. To control for assay variability, the measurement of the initial sample in which molecular relapse was suspected should be included during the analysis of a repeat sample. Due to cost constraints, reference laboratories may not store or retest previous patient specimens. Specific laboratory practices should be carefully considered when selecting a testing platform for individual patients. Furthermore, quantitative standards should be included that cover the CT (cycle threshold) range of the patient sample to ensure linearity of the assay at the appropriate measured MRD level [19]. Again, for cost-containment, commercial laboratories may select to routinely run only a very small set of quantitative standards, covering a very narrow CT and linear range.

High precaution should be taken when interpreting *BCR-ABL1* RQ-PCR results at the time of diagnosis, particularly if the assay employed is being performed only in single-well reactions. Very low levels of *BCR-ABL1* mRNA have been reported in healthy individuals [20, 21]. Therefore, low-positive findings by a testing facility utilizing a platform designed for "deep molecular remission" testing may not be sufficient for the diagnosis of CML. Reference laboratories releasing low-positive BCR/ABL1 test results for specimens with unknown clinical history should take precaution and either 1) confirm that CML (or ALL) has indeed been previously diagnosed and the patient has been treated or 2) inform the clinician or pathologist that low-level *BCR-ABL1* transcript levels are not in keeping with a diagnostic presentation.

PML-RARA

Acute promyelocytic leukemia (APL) is characterized by the t(15;17)(q22;q21) translocation. The *PML-RARA* fusion gene transcripts are the molecular result of this chromosomal rearrangement and can be quantified by "real-time" quantitative reverse transcriptase polymerase chain reaction (RQ-PCR). There are three possible *PML-RARA* isoforms, referred to as long (L or bcr1), variant (V or bcr2), and short (S or bcr3). The chimeric PML-RARA protein is considered as a transcriptional repressor, which binds to DNA in the absence of its ligand (retinoic acid, RA) [18]. An important MRD endpoint at the end of consolidation treatment, after all-trans retinoic acid (ATRA) with chemotherapy or with arsenic trioxide, is the achievement of PCR negativity [19]. A change of *PML-RARA* PCR status from undetectable to detectable in either bone marrow (BM) or peripheral blood (PB) is considered an indicator for imminent disease relapse after confirmation by a repeat specimen [22].

Monitoring testing of BM or PB in 3-month intervals has been recommended, in order to detect molecular relapse. Whereas *PML-RARA* RQ-PCR protocols have been outlined in detail by EAC (Europe Against Cancer program) [18], uniform assay guidelines to standardize quantification are still lacking. It has to be noted that patient-specific monitoring designs are of the utmost importance. In contrast to *BCR-ABL1*, *PML-RARA* transcripts vary greatly between patients at the time of diagnosis. In order to accurately quantify percent and log reduction rates during the course of treatment, side-by-side testing of the previous patient specimens is required. When selecting or establishing a laboratory for *PML-RARA* quantitative monitoring, it is important to verify that testing algorithms do not rely solely on commercial, cell line, or plasmid standards. In order to reduce intrinsic assay variation, storage and retesting of previous patient specimens are pertinent. In addition, it is crucial that diagnostic bone marrow and peripheral blood specimens are collected before treatment and archived for RNA/cDNA within 72 h for *PML-RARA* RQ-PCR. Only the availability of patient-specific baseline specimens will allow for accurate monitoring results. Whereas *BCR-ABL1* and other RQ-PCR platforms can miss variant translocations only detectable by FISH and/or cytogenetic analysis limiting their applicability during a diagnostic workup, *PML-RARA* RQ-PCR has proven itself an excellent screening tool. Fast RQ-PCR platforms can give results in less than an hour, facilitating rapid diagnosis and treatment intervention to reduce bleeding complications in APL. In addition, the detection of the *PML-RARA* fusion transcripts by PCR has been demonstrated in variant APL cases characterized by cryptic translocations or small insertion events undetectable by conventional FISH and cytogenetic testing [23, 24].

CBF-AML (Core-Binding Factor AML)

Recurrent genetic abnormalities in acute myeloid leukemia (AML) are associated with distinctive clinicopathological features as well as prognostic subcategories [25]. The balanced chromosomal rearrangements t(8;21) and inv(16) or t(16;16) are considered as evidence for AML regardless of blast cell counts. The core-binding factor (CBF) transcription factor is essential for hematopoiesis. Both heterodimeric components of CBF, RUNX1 (also called AML1 and CBFA) and CBFB, are implicated in chromosomal translocations of CBF-AML (core-binding factor AML). These rearrangements create fusion genes encoding chimeric proteins implicated in leukemogenesis. Whereas agreement between RQ-PCR and multiparameter flow cytometry (MFC) is known to be weak in CBF-AML, the two technologies are considered complementary to each other [26]. Discrepancies between the two technologies can occur since molecular fusion transcripts may exist in nondividing cells or dying cells immediately after high-dose chemotherapy. Low levels of core-binding factor fusion transcripts may also persist and are considered compatible with durable remission. MFC sensitivity can be affected by the frequent myelomonocytic immunophenotype in CBF-AML. Monocytic blasts can exhibit significant overlap with normal/regenerating monocytes, creating a challenge for MRD detection by MFC. Therefore, preemptive treatment regardless of MFC findings may be considered when rising RQ-PCR levels are encountered for serial monitoring specimens [19].

t(8;21); RUNX1-RUNX1T1

AML with t(8;21)(q22;q22.1) resulting in *RUNX1-RUNX1T1* fusion transcripts has been associated with favorable long-term outcome. Quantification of *RUNX1-RUNX1T1* transcript values is considered a valuable tool to monitor treatment [27, 28]. Achievement of >3 log reduction rates in bone marrow has been associated with better outcome [19]. Similar to *PML-RARA*, collection and storage of diagnostic specimens are of utmost importance. Individual *RUNX1-RUNX1T1* transcript levels at diagnosis may vary greatly from patient to patient. Whereas plasmid standards are commercially available to assist quantification, they cannot be used as surrogate baselines to determine patient-specific reduction rates in the absence of diagnostic material. *RUNX1-RUNX1T1* RQ-PCR protocols have been published by EAC [18], however standardization among laboratories is currently not common practice. The comparison of copy number values from laboratory to laboratory, or comparison to published clinical studies, should be interpreted with caution. In order to achieve clinically meaningful results, individual patients should be consistently monitored by one laboratory. An important difference has to be noted for *RUNX1-RUNX1T1* in comparison to *BCR-ABL1* or *PML-RARA* monitoring approaches: low levels of *RUNX1-RUNX1T1* transcript values may be detectable by PCR for years after initial diagnosis. As a possible explanation, t(8;21) has been detected in non-progenitor cell populations (e.g., mast cells), and low level of fusion transcripts may not always accurately reflect residual disease status [29].

Therefore, stable, low levels of *RUNX1-RUNX1T1* values have to be carefully correlated to other clinical findings, particularly flow cytometry MRD. Flow cytometric cell sorting (FACS) can present itself as a valuable clinical tool to determine if t(8;21) is indeed present in the progenitor cell fractions or lingering in mature compartments (e.g., mast cells). Please refer to Subsection "FACS-FISH (Fluorescence In Situ Hybridization)" for FACS-FISH.

Inv(16)

Inv(16) or the rarer t(16;16)(p13;q22) leads to fusion of the CBFB chain gene with the smooth muscle myosin heavy chain gene MYH11. The resulting fusion transcripts present themselves as a suitable molecular marker for both diagnostic and monitoring studies. 10 different types of *CBFB-MYH11* transcripts have been reported. Type A, D and E represent approximately 95% of all cases, and can be detected using the EAC protocol design [18]. It is pertinent that a diagnostic specimen is analyzed within 72 h. This practice will not only establish a patient-specific baseline value but also ensure that the RQ-PCR platform of choice can indeed be used for monitoring purposes. Quantitative MRD monitoring using *CBFB-MYH11* RQ-PCR is recommended by the 2018 guidelines [19]. Similar to *RUNX1-RUNX1T1*, it has to be noted that low, stable levels of transcripts may be detectable for extended periods of time without evidence of disease relapse. FACS-FISH strategies can be implemented to investigate inv(16) status of progenitor versus other mature cell compartments [please refer to Subsection "FACS-FISH (Fluorescence In Situ Hybridization)" FACS-FISH]. Standardization of copy number or percent positivity values among different laboratories is still suboptimal. Comparisons of quantitative values among different laboratories or comparisons to published cutoff values have to be interpreted with caution. Patient-specific monitoring approaches (individual log and percent reduction rates) can be performed in a quantitative fashion if diagnostic materials have been analyzed and archived. A single laboratory should be chosen for continuous monitoring of individual patients. Several selection criteria should be considered: (1) international standards and assay design according to EAC [18]; (2) archiving of diagnostic and monitoring specimens; (3) routine side-by-side studies of diagnostic and monitoring specimens for accurate and patient-specific quantification; (4) triplicate testing; (5) Ct values of standard curve in the linear range of the patient specimen; (6) fast turnaround times without test batching; (7) lower level of detection; (8) correlation to flow cytometry MRD findings; and (9) FACS-FISH for confirmation studies, if indicated [30, 31].

MLL

MLL (KMT2A, 11q23) can be rearranged with dozens of various chromosomal translocation partners. Breakpoints can vary over multiple intronic sequences, complicating assay design. DNA-based approaches have been used for breakpoint identification [32], and the MLL recombinome has been characterized in acute leukemia [33]. Whereas a total of

135 different MLL rearrangements have been identified, only 9 specific gene fusions account for more than 90% of recombinations of the MLL gene. Monitoring for a vast majority of fusions has been described. Assay platforms most commonly available in a clinical laboratory setting are *MLL-AF4* (4;11) [18], *MLL-AF9* t(9;11) [34], *MLL-ENL/ELL* t(11;19) [35, 36], *MLL-AF10* t(10;11) [37, 38], and *MLL-AF1* t(1;11) RQ-PCR [39–41].

Establishment of MLL translocation-specific PCR primers for MRD analyses for all patients is the goal. Standardization of quantification protocols, as well as side-by-side analysis of patient-specific baseline specimens, has to be considered for each design.

WT1 Expression

WT1 expression is only recommended as a monitoring assay if no other MRD markers are available in the patient [19]. A validated *WT1* MRD assay design has been published by ELN [42]. The Wilms tumor gene WT1 is overexpressed in most patients with AML. Its utility for MRD monitoring has been viewed as controversial, which may have been a reflection of a variety of assay designs being used. However, the application of a standardized *WT1* assay has been proven to provide an independent prognostic marker for monitoring purposes [42]. Since *WT1* expression is not leukemia-specific, extensive studies of normal specimens are necessary to establish levels of expression and cutoff values. Both copy number standards as well as side-by-side studies of patient baseline specimens for quantification by the ΔCt method have to be employed. Specimen testing has to be performed in triplicates. Instrument settings including thresholds for Ct (cycle threshold) value determination have to be defined. Stringent criteria for RNA input as well as RNA integrity have to be established. Whereas pretreatment *WT1* expression levels are not predictive of outcome, the kinetics of *WT1* transcript reduction can provide a key prognostic factor. Failure to normalize *WT1* transcript levels by post-consolidation can distinguish a patient group with increased risk for relapse.

BCL1 and BCL2 RQ-PCR

Two types of non-Hodgkin's lymphoma (NHL) are characterized by specific chromosomal translocations. The t(14;18) (q32;q21.3) is characteristic for follicular lymphoma, whereas t(11;14)(q13;q32) is the hallmark of mantle cell lymphoma. These translocations can serve as tumor-associated DNA markers. Both the t(14;18) and t(11;14) real-time PCR assays are used to quantitate minimal residual disease (MRD) [43]. The use of polymerase chain reaction (PCR) to detect rearrangement of the BCL2 gene has successfully been used to detect molecular responses predicting clinical response in follicular lymphoma clinical trials [44]. Quantitative real-time polymerase chain reaction (PCR) assay designs with specific primers for the *BCL2* MBR-JH and the BCL2 mcr-JH rearrangement as well as *BCL1* MTC-JH rearrangement regions are available by the BIOMED-2 Concerted Action protocol [45]. These assays can detect amplifiable t(14;18) or t(11;14) translocations with a sensitivity of at least 1 in 10^4 cells (0.01%). It is important to note that a negative result does not exclude the presence of t(14;18) or t(11;14) translocations. Only approximately 50% of t(11;14) translocations and approximately 70% of t(14;18) can be detected by PCR. The lack of detectable amplification by RQ-PCR in a diagnostic specimen indicates that these assays cannot be used to monitor minimal residual disease in a particular patient. The analysis and procurement of diagnostic specimens is crucial to utilize BCL1 or BCL2 RQ-PCR for monitoring purposes. Alternate methods for patients with non-amplifiable BCL1/BCL2 breakpoints have to be established. Clonal Immunoglobulin gene rearrangement sequences detected at the time of diagnosis can be utilized for FACS-PCR (see section "FACS Immunoglobulin (Ig) and T-Cell Receptor (TCR) Gene Rearrangements") or NGS monitoring approaches (see section "B- and T-Cell Malignancies").

New Emerging and Patient-Specific

Unfortunately, conventional leukemia-specific translocations suitable for RQ-PCR monitoring are only available in a portion of patients [2]. With the advent of next-generation sequencing, the identification rate of novel and/or unique fusion transcripts is increasing, e.g., Ph-like B-ALL or pediatric AML [82]. Flexible RQ-PCR platforms and customizable designs for molecules suitable as quantitative standards have to be established for fast-track clinical assay validation. As efforts for personalized assay designs increase, new emerging fusion transcripts have and will become available for clinical use. For example, *CBFA2T3-GLIS2* fusion transcripts, which are the molecular result of the cryptic chromosome 16 inversion [inv (16)(p13.3q24.3)], are associated with a poor prognosis in pediatric AML [46] or *NPM1-MLF1* t(3;5) fusion transcripts, which are the molecular result of the rare t(3;5) (q25;q35) translocation, which is associated with myelodysplastic syndrome (MDS), often prior to AML. The incidence of t(3;5)(q25;q35) is seen in approximately 0.5% of patients with AML and is observed in all age groups but more commonly in younger patients [47, 48]. Another example is *NUP98/NSD1* fusion transcripts, the results of a cryptic t(5;11) translocation in acute myeloid leukemia (AML) [49, 50]. The list of defined fusion transcripts is growing and their detection at diagnosis is being optimized with advances in RNA sequencing. Universally applicable protocols for standardized RQ-PCR platforms have to be established, in order to provide reliable quantitative detection methods for the majority of patients.

Flow Cytometric Cell Sorting (FACS)

FACS in combination with subsequent molecular analysis can increase sensitivity of MRD findings. Linking immunophenotype with genotype is also a powerful tool to provide testing specificity as well as clinical confidence. Its application can range from making confident calls in the absence of a diagnostic specimen to distinguishing (a) re-generating bone marrow progenitors from low-level disease; (b) reactive side-clones from original leukemic processes; (c) persistent chromosomal rearrangements or gene mutations in non-leukemic components from true residual disease. In addition, we have previously demonstrated the application of this approach to discern genetic properties as well as relationships of co-existing clonal processes [51–53].

Furthermore, sub-groups of ALL with CML-like biology can be identified by determining which cell lineages carry t(9;22) at diagnosis [54, 55]. This chapter will focus on the utility of FACS for residual disease confirmation, while excluding STR analysis in bone marrow transplant settings, described elsewhere.

FACS Immunoglobulin (Ig) and T-Cell Receptor (TCR) Gene Rearrangements

Ig and TCR gene rearrangements are frequently used as targets in PCR-based MRD studies [56–59]. These rearrangements can be considered as "fingerprints" for lymphoid cells since each clone has its own deletions and random insertion of nucleotides at the junction sites of the gene segments. A clonal leukemic cell population of lymphoid origin can be detected by the presence of a strong signal for a single gene rearrangement of a specific size after multiplex PCR amplification, whereas a polyclonal lymphocyte population results in uniform Gaussian distribution of amplicons. In order to use these gene rearrangements for MRD analysis by real-time PCR, patient-specific assays can be created after sequencing the gene rearrangement amplicon. Several studies have compared the sensitivity in MRD detection of flow cytometry and molecular approaches [60–64].

Flow cytometric-based immunophenotyping provides a rapid and sensitive method for detecting up to one leukemic cell in 10^4 normal cells. Molecular analysis of gene rearrangements can routinely detect a minimum of 1 monoclonal B cell in 1000 normal cells using immunoglobulin heavy (IgH) chain multiplex assays and 1 monoclonal T cell in 100 normal cells using TCR gamma (TCRG) primer sets. Patient-specific real-time quantitative PCR (RQ-PCR) assays can be established for Ig/TCR gene rearrangements with sensitivities ranging from 0.01% to 0.001%, but assay setup is currently too time-consuming for a routine clinical application. Next-generation sequencing (NGS) of Ig and TCR targets may provide a more broadly accessible testing platform for MRD assessment (please refer to section "B- and T-Cell Malignancies"). In a previous study, we demonstrated a two-step technique for detecting and confirming low levels of disease by integrating phenotype analysis using standardized flow cytometry panels, cell sorting, and subsequent genotype analysis using multiplex gene rearrangement PCR [65]. DNA was amplified using the Biomed-2 [45]. Primer sets for the IgH chain region of framework 1, 2, and 3 for the detection of clonal B-cell proliferations. To identify T-cell clonality, a TCRG gene rearrangement assay was used. PCR amplicons were analyzed by fluorescence detection using a capillary electrophoresis sequencer. Our study showed that combining cell sorting with clonality profiling effectively lowered sensitivity limits for disease detection and was also able to provide independent confirmation of the tumor detection without the need for patient-specific assay designs. Patient specimens with small abnormal B-lymphoid populations or with small aberrant T-cell populations as detected by flow cytometry were analyzed by (IgH) or TCRG gene rearrangement PCR with and without cell purification to illustrate the utility of relating aberrant phenotype to a specific genotype for several clinical applications. This approach can be useful in a bone marrow transplant setting where the patient is often first encountered when in remission. The detection of MRD is illustrated for a precursor B-lineage (pre-B-ALL), post-hematopoietic stem cell transplant. Upon analysis of the bone marrow, 0.05% abnormal lymphoblasts were detected by flow cytometry, expressing HLA-DR, bright CD10, dim CD19, and bright CD34, but lacking expression of CD45. No monoclonal or polyclonal signal was detected by the IgH gene rearrangement assay in this bone marrow specimen due to the presence of very few normal B cells (0.02% / data not shown). The small abnormal lymphoblast population was sorted using a CD10+ and CD45- gate (Fig. 3.2a) and analyzed for B-cell clonality by PCR. B-cell gene rearrangement PCR alone can be used to assess and monitor clonality if the suspected malignant population is present at a level of approximately 1%. To increase sensitivity for minimal residual disease monitoring, the use of allele-specific (ASO) primers in combination with germline (Jg) primers and (Jg) TaqMan probes have been shown as a useful tool with a sensitivity of 0.01 (10^{-4}) to a maximum of 0.001% (10^{-5}) [56–58, 66, 67].

Quantification of patient-specific Ig/TCR rearrangements has been standardized by the EuroMRD international network [57, 58, 68, 69].

However, in many cases those sensitivities cannot be reached due to nonspecific amplification of gene rearrangements in the normal lymphocytes present. After treatment, the background of normal B and T cells may be particularly high, lowering the sensitivity even further. In addition to the cumbersome setup of patient-specific assays, several gene rearrangement loci should be used simultaneously as PCR targets, since single rearrangements are unstable and can be lost during clonal transformation and following disease relapse due to continuing gene rearrangements or further gene deletions. In particular, for malignancies demonstrating oligoclonality with

---

FIGURE 3.2 A small abnormal population of cells was detected by flow cytometry in the bone marrow from a patient with precursor B acute lymphoblastic leukemia after hematopoietic stem cell transplant. The cell fraction in the rectangle was sorted using a CD10+ and CD45- gate (**a**) for B-cell gene rearrangement studies. Molecular analysis of unseparated bone marrow showed no distinct monoclonality profile (**b**). The sorted tumor cell population demonstrated a monoclonal peak profile (**c**) with amplicons for IgH framework regions one (FR1), two (FR2), and three (FR3). The identical monoclonality profile was found in subsequent monitoring specimens with confirmed minimal residual disease. (Data not shown)

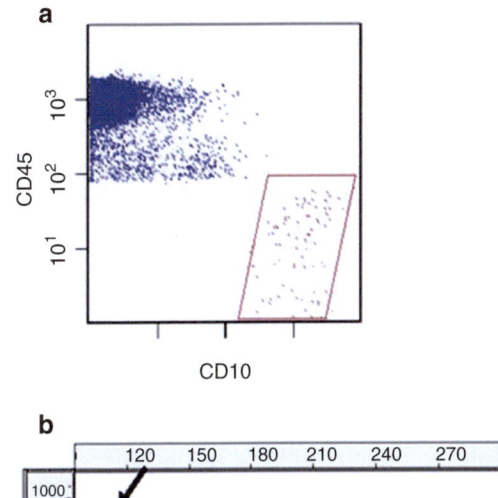
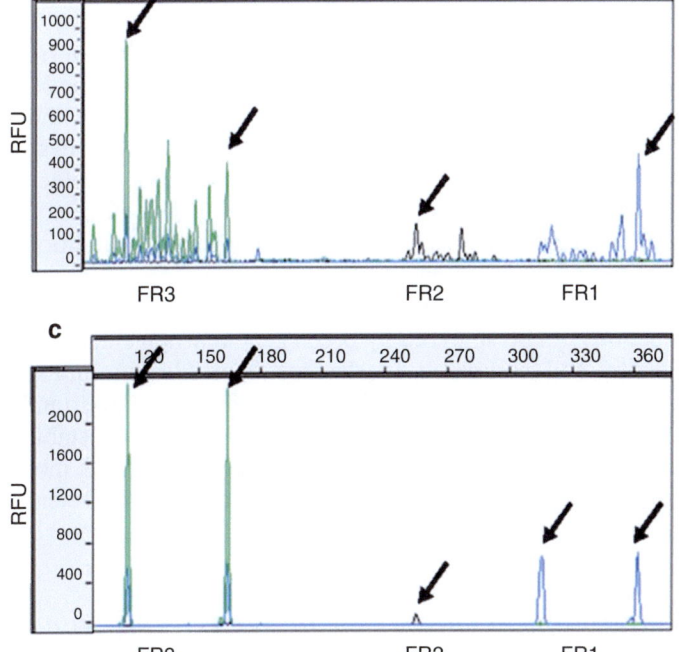

multiple subclones present at diagnosis, the likelihood of losing a PCR target during follow-up is significantly increased [59]. Combining routine immunophenotyping with cell purification and subsequent gene rearrangement studies by multifluorescent PCR and capillary electrophoresis analysis, the presence of a monoclonal leukemic cell population can be confirmed and lowers the assay sensitivity level. Suspicious cell populations down to levels of 0.01% can be identified and purified by flow cytometry. Subsequent gene rearrangement analysis can confirm the identity of putative monoclonal peaks in reference to the unsorted specimen and/or to the original clone from a diagnostic specimen or paraffin-embedded tumor biopsy. The combination of the two technologies allows the identification of a clonogenic neoplastic cell population which would be undetectable or inconclusive by conventional analysis. For minimal disease, monitoring the amplicon size of the clonal gene rearrangement, known from a previous diagnostic marrow aspirate or paraffin-embedded biopsy specimen, becomes the tumor-specific marker without the need to develop patient-specific DNA primers, probes, or antibody panels. This approach could also be applicable to demonstrate that a suspicious phenotype is not monoclonal and/or recurrent disease, thus preventing potential additional chemotherapy for the patient.

In addition, CD138-enriched or CD38-sorted plasma cell fractions can be analyzed by B-cell gene rearrangement PCR studies and compared to diagnostic profiles in multiple myeloma or other plasma cell neoplasms. Most importantly, this approach can also be useful to confirm and establish clone-specific Ig/TC-sequences for subsequent NGS monitoring studies in all lymphoid malignancies (please refer to section "B- and T-Cell Malignancies").

FACS-FISH (Fluorescence In Situ Hybridization)

Residual disease monitoring by flow cytometry in AML has gained increasing clinical significance in recent years. Two analysis concepts, namely, "leukemia-associated immunophenotype (LAIP)" and "difference from normal," have been successfully used to monitor treatment response and predict clinical outcome. The LAIP approach to detect residual disease presupposes that the phenotype identified at diagnosis remains constant after therapy. AML differs from other hematopoietic neoplasms with respect to the increased phenotypic heterogeneity observed within the leukemic clone, reported in pediatric [70] as well as adult patients [71]. Diagnostic and relapse phenotypes can differ up to 80% of the time. If the phenotype changes following chemotherapy, particularly if new antigens appear or antigens disappear, detection of residual disease can be challenging [72]. A "difference from normal approach" using multidimensional flow cytometry allows for a comprehensive analysis of the heterogeneous cell populations that can be observed in acute myeloid leukemia [1]. "Difference from normal" is independent of the phenotype of the abnormal cell population. There is no requirement for access to the diagnostic phenotype since the flow cytometry assay focuses on the positions of the normal regenerating cells.

FACS-FISH can provide important specificity for residual disease confirmation in AML patients with unknown or shifting immunophenotype. By enriching or purifying the myeloblast population with subsequent testing for chromosome aberrations, the presence of neoplastic cells can be confirmed (Fig. 3.3). FACS-FISH can reveal the presence of neoplastic cells harboring chromosomal aberrations in the myeloblast compartment. These findings can confirm the presence of residual leukemia. Combining an aberrant or suspicious immunophenotype with chromosome analysis can significantly increase clinical specificity. Confidence in testing specificity is important when monitoring treatment of neoplastic processes with increasingly sensitive assay platforms. Positive results may trigger therapeutic intervention with associated morbidity and mortality. Therefore, false-positive results must be avoided at all cost. Interdisciplinary integration of flow cytometry and fluorescence in situ hybridization can achieve that goal. Confidence in low-level findings can be acquired by confirmatory testing of the cells in question (Fig. 3.3).

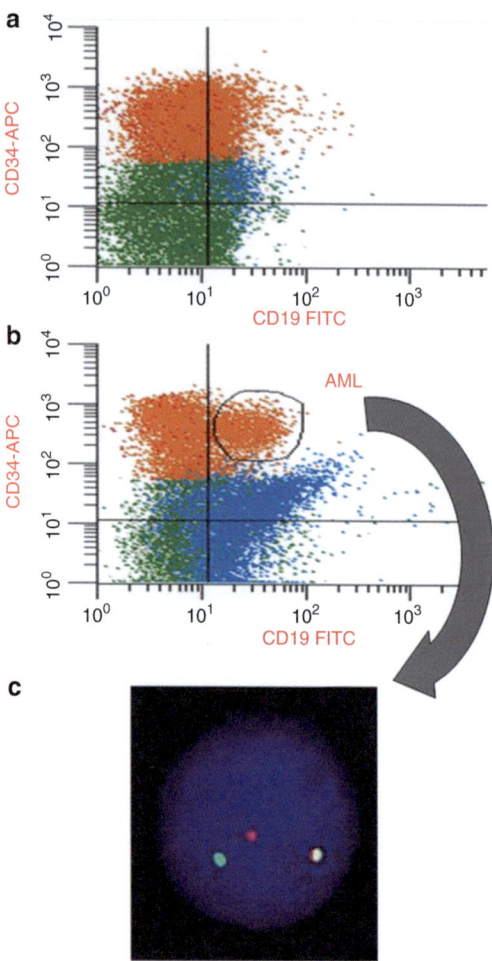

FIGURE 3.3 An AML specimen with t(11;19) exhibited low proportions of abnormal progenitor cells (CD34 +, orange) as well as abnormal maturing monocytes (light blue) at diagnosis (**a**). After the first cycle of induction chemotherapy, an abnormal myeloid progenitor cell population expressing CD19 was detected at 0.5% (**b**). The CD19 positive population was sorted for fluorescence in situ hybridization studies revealing 95% harboring a rearranged MLL (KMT2A, 11q23) gene locus (**c**)

In addition, specificity of molecular testing results can also be improved by FACS-FISH. For example, flow cytometric findings and RQ-PCR findings do not always correlate in CBF-AML [please refer to section "CBF-AML (Core-Binding Factor AML)"]. Detecting and confirming the presence of RUNX1/RUNX1T1 or CBFB rearrangements in non-leukemic cells can help interpret the discrepant results [29]. Chromosomal translocations may linger in mature cell compartments (e.g., mast cells) and thereby cause persistent low-level fusion transcript findings without the presence of residual leukemia (Fig. 3.4).

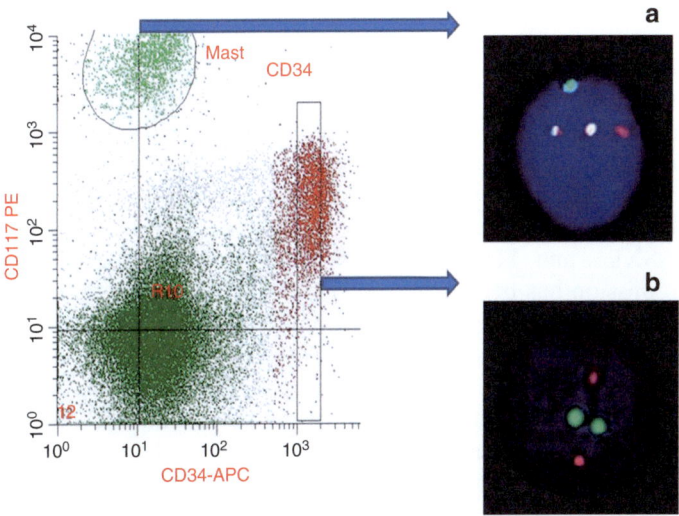

FIGURE 3.4 FACS-FISH analysis of a bone marrow aspirate of an AML with t(8;21) after treatment. Flow cytometry showed no evidence of residual AML. *RUNX1/RUNX1T1* RQ-PCR was positive. Flow cytometric cell sorting was used to analyze the mast cell (CD117) as well as progenitor cell (CD34) fraction for the presence of t(8;21) by FISH. FACS-FISH revealed the presence of double RUNX1/RUNX1T1 fusions (1R1G2F signal pattern) in the mast cell population (**a**), whereas the cells collected in the CD34 progenitor gate did not reveal the translocation (2R2G signal pattern) (**b**)

NGS (Next-Generation Sequencing)

Recent developments in NGS have attracted much attention for its use in monitoring residual disease. Enhanced sensitivity levels are foreseen if specific target molecules can be identified and a sufficient number of cells are analyzed. Whereas NGS is slowly emerging in routine clinical practice for monitoring purposes, standardization of protocols still has to be achieved. Quality and sensitivity controls, defined specimen requirements, as well as bioinformatics guidelines have to be implemented to ensure reliable results [73].

AML

Patients without the presence of known fusion transcripts for RQ-PCR monitoring may present with gene mutations at the time of diagnosis by NGS. Care has to be taken to discern mutations that may not accurately reflect disease status from markers that can reliably be used for MRD monitoring [19]. Preleukemic founder clone mutations (e.g., DNMT3A, ASXL1, and TET2) may persist at significant levels after remission has been achieved [74–76]. Moreover, these mutations may also occur in healthy individuals and increase in frequency with age [77]. This newly discovered phenomenon has been named clonal hematopoiesis of indeterminate potential (CHIP) but is currently limited to mutations identified at allele frequencies of ≥2%. Combining aberrant immunophenotype information with genotype analysis by flow cytometric cell sorting (please refer to section "Flow Cytometric Cell Sorting (FACS)") can improve specificity of mutation findings in a monitoring setting. The use and monitoring of several markers can also help overcome limitations due to clonal heterogeneity and CHIP. However, several AML-related gene mutations can also be found as germline mutations. Whereas they may increase the risk of AML development, they cannot be used as monitoring markers. A variant allele frequency (VAF) of ~50% may be an indicator that germline origin has to be excluded. Furthermore, the sensitivity range of current routine NGS approaches is only ~1%, which is inadequate for assessing deep molecular response. Recent developments in error-corrected NGS may help overcome sensitivity limitations [78]. Flow cytometric cell sorting of suspicious progenitors or alternatively patient-specific leukemic progenitors with subsequent NGS analysis can improve both sensitivity as well as specificity of testing results.

B- and T-Cell Malignancies

Ig or TCR gene rearrangements represent unique genetic markers or molecular signatures (DNA fingerprint) for B- and T-cell malignancies. PCR-based high-throughput sequencing (HTS) (or also known as NGS) of Ig/TCR rearrangements has gained attention as an attractive option for MRD monitoring in B- and T-cell malignancies [79, 80]. In contrast to RQ-PCR approaches, the labor-intensive identification of clone-specific Ig/TCR targets with subsequent patient-specific assay design can be avoided. As additional advantage, NGS/HTS Ig/TCR may also be able to detect ongoing clonal evolution or the emergence of subclones. Furthermore, early time point results are possible since time-consuming ASO-RQ-PCR design and validations can be avoided. Multiplex PCR with multiple primer sets are used to amplify all potential rearrangements in a sample. Consequently, the correct rearrangement sequence has to be identified. Arbitrary cutoffs to identify the clonal rearrangements can be error-prone. Unrelated B- or T-cell expansions may be misinterpreted as malignancy-specific rearrangements. This pitfall particularly arises when the applied primer set does amplify the rearrangements of the targeted malignancy. Somatic hypermutation of Ig loci as well as oligoclonality at diagnosis can be the underlying causes. This conundrum can be avoided if a diagnostic sample is carefully analyzed. Classic Sanger sequencing can be employed to identify the correct Ig/TCR fingerprint of the index clone at the time of diagnosis. If specificity of a clonal rearrangement is in question (e.g., no dominant appearance in the Ig or TCR gene rearrangement assessment), FACS studies with subsequent molecular analysis can be used to identify the correct clonotype [51]. When evaluating the sensitivity level of NGS/HTS Ig/TCR studies, one has to consider the cellular DNA input. A sensitivity of 10^{-6} can only be reached if the input DNA equals one million cells per sequencing reaction [81]. Availability of sufficient DNA may be challenging in specimens with low cellularity collected subsequent to treatment. In addition to leukemia, Ig/TCR-specific detection by HTS/NGS can also be utilized for bone marrow staging, as well as residual disease monitoring of non-Hodgkin's lymphoma and plasma cell neoplasms. Again, the confirmation of the correct clonotype in a diagnostic specimen is fundamental for monitoring findings with reliable specificity.

In summary, the predictive power of residual disease monitoring for hematopoietic malignancies is undisputed. However, technical pitfalls and challenges have to be taken into consideration to avoid false-positive or false-negative interpretations. In-depth understanding of the technologies used and most importantly their inherent limitations is crucial for accurate clinical associations. Standardizations of high complexity testing modalities are challenging, particularly with the continuous evolution of technical platforms. Ongoing inter- and intra-laboratory validations have to be performed. For that purpose, defined clinical specimen sets as well as correlation to outcome data have to be made available to clinical reference laboratories.

References

1. Loken MR, Alonzo TA, Pardo L, Gerbing RB, Raimondi SC, Hirsch BA, et al. Residual disease detected by multidimensional flow cytometry signifies high relapse risk in patients with de novo acute myeloid leukemia: a report from Children's oncology group. Blood. 2012;120(8):1581–8.
2. Szczepanski T, Orfao A, van der Velden VH, San Miguel JF, van Dongen JJ. Minimal residual disease in leukaemia patients. Lancet Oncol. 2001;2(7):409–17.

3. van Dongen JJ, Seriu T, Panzer-Grumayer ER, Biondi A, Pongers-Willemse MJ, Corral L, et al. Prognostic value of minimal residual disease in acute lymphoblastic leukaemia in childhood. Lancet. 1998;352(9142):1731–8.
4. Wood B, Wu D, Crossley B, Dai Y, Williamson D, Gawad C, et al. Measurable residual disease detection by high-throughput sequencing improves risk stratification for pediatric B-ALL. Blood. 2018;131(12):1350–9.
5. Berry DA, Zhou S, Higley H, Mukundan L, Fu S, Reaman GH, et al. Association of Minimal Residual Disease with Clinical Outcome in pediatric and adult acute lymphoblastic leukemia: a meta-analysis. JAMA Oncol. 2017;3(7):e170580.
6. Radich J, Ladne P, Gooley T. Polymerase chain reaction-based detection of minimal residual disease in acute lymphoblastic leukemia predicts relapse after allogeneic BMT. Biol Blood Marrow Transplant. 1995;1(1):24–31.
7. Hoshino A, Funato T, Munakata Y, Ishii T, Abe S, Ishizawa K, et al. Detection of clone-specific immunoglobulin heavy chain genes in the bone marrow of B-cell-lineage lymphoma after treatment. Tohoku J Exp Med. 2004;203(3):155–64.
8. Terwijn M, van Putten WL, Kelder A, van der Velden VH, Brooimans RA, Pabst T, et al. High prognostic impact of flow cytometric minimal residual disease detection in acute myeloid leukemia: data from the HOVON/SAKK AML 42A study. J Clin Oncol. 2013;31(31):3889–97.
9. Walter RB, Buckley SA, Pagel JM, Wood BL, Storer BE, Sandmaier BM, et al. Significance of minimal residual disease before myeloablative allogeneic hematopoietic cell transplantation for AML in first and second complete remission. Blood. 2013;122(10):1813–21.
10. Buccisano F, Maurillo L, Del Principe MI, Del Poeta G, Sconocchia G, Lo-Coco F, et al. Prognostic and therapeutic implications of minimal residual disease detection in acute myeloid leukemia. Blood. 2012;119(2):332–41.
11. Bradfield SM, Radich JP, Loken MR. Graft-versus-leukemia effect in acute lymphoblastic leukemia: the importance of tumor burden and early detection. Leukemia. 2004;18(6):1156–8.
12. Szczepanski T. Why and how to quantify minimal residual disease in acute lymphoblastic leukemia? Leukemia. 2007;21(4):622–6.
13. Branford S. Molecular monitoring in chronic myeloid leukemia-how low can you go? Hematology Am Soc Hematol Educ Program. 2016;2016(1):156–63.

14. Beillard E, Pallisgaard N, van der Velden VH, Bi W, Dee R, van der Schoot E, et al. Evaluation of candidate control genes for diagnosis and residual disease detection in leukemic patients using 'real-time' quantitative reverse-transcriptase polymerase chain reaction (RQ-PCR) - a Europe against cancer program. Leukemia. 2003;17(12):2474–86.
15. Cross NC, White HE, Colomer D, Ehrencrona H, Foroni L, Gottardi E, et al. Laboratory recommendations for scoring deep molecular responses following treatment for chronic myeloid leukemia. Leukemia. 2015;29(5):999–1003.
16. Cross NC, White HE, Muller MC, Saglio G, Hochhaus A. Standardized definitions of molecular response in chronic myeloid leukemia. Leukemia. 2012;26(10):2172–5.
17. Hughes TP, Saglio G, Kantarjian HM, Guilhot F, Niederwieser D, Rosti G, et al. Early molecular response predicts outcomes in patients with chronic myeloid leukemia in chronic phase treated with frontline nilotinib or imatinib. Blood. 2014;123(9):1353–60.
18. Gabert J, Beillard E, van der Velden VH, Bi W, Grimwade D, Pallisgaard N, et al. Standardization and quality control studies of 'real-time' quantitative reverse transcriptase polymerase chain reaction of fusion gene transcripts for residual disease detection in leukemia - a Europe against Cancer program. Leukemia. 2003;17(12):2318–57.
19. Schuurhuis GJ, Heuser M, Freeman S, Bene MC, Buccisano F, Cloos J, et al. Minimal/measurable residual disease in AML: a consensus document from the European LeukemiaNet MRD working party. Blood. 2018;131(12):1275–91.
20. Biernaux C, Loos M, Sels A, Huez G, Stryckmans P. Detection of major bcr-abl gene expression at a very low level in blood cells of some healthy individuals. Blood. 1995;86(8):3118–22.
21. Bose S, Deininger M, Gora-Tybor J, Goldman JM, Melo JV. The presence of typical and atypical BCR-ABL fusion genes in leukocytes of normal individuals: biologic significance and implications for the assessment of minimal residual disease. Blood. 1998;92(9):3362–7.
22. Grimwade D, Jovanovic JV, Hills RK, Nugent EA, Patel Y, Flora R, et al. Prospective minimal residual disease monitoring to predict relapse of acute promyelocytic leukemia and to direct pre-emptive arsenic trioxide therapy. J Clin Oncol. 2009;27(22):3650–8.
23. Welch JS, Westervelt P, Ding L, Larson DE, Klco JM, Kulkarni S, et al. Use of whole-genome sequencing to diagnose a cryptic fusion oncogene. JAMA. 2011;305(15):1577–84.

24. Koshy J, Qian YW, Bhagwath G, Willis M, Kelley TW, Papenhausen P. Microarray, gene sequencing, and reverse transcriptase-polymerase chain reaction analyses of a cryptic PML-RARA translocation. Cancer Genet. 2012;205(10): 537–40.
25. Swerdlow SHCE, Harris NL, Jaffe ES, Pileri SA, Stein H, Thiele J, editors. WHO classification of tumours of haematopoietic and lymphoid tissues: International Agency for Research on Cancer; 2017.
26. Ouyang J, Goswami M, Peng J, Zuo Z, Daver N, Borthakur G, et al. Comparison of multiparameter flow cytometry Immunophenotypic analysis and quantitative RT-PCR for the detection of minimal residual disease of Core binding factor acute myeloid leukemia. Am J Clin Pathol. 2016;145(6):769–77.
27. Tobal K, Newton J, Macheta M, Chang J, Morgenstern G, Evans PA, et al. Molecular quantitation of minimal residual disease in acute myeloid leukemia with t(8;21) can identify patients in durable remission and predict clinical relapse. Blood. 2000;95(3):815–9.
28. Wang Y, Wu DP, Liu QF, Qin YZ, Wang JB, Xu LP, et al. In adults with t(8;21)AML, posttransplant RUNX1/RUNX1T1-based MRD monitoring, rather than c-KIT mutations, allows further risk stratification. Blood. 2014;124(12):1880–6.
29. Dong ZM, Ramakrishnan A, Chauncey TR, Loken MR, Zehentner BK, Wu DY et al. No adverse effect of residual neoplastic mast cells in systemic Mastocytosis associated with acute myeloid leukemia with T(8;21) (Q22;Q22); Runx1-Runx1t1 after bone marrow transplantation. Ann Clin Pathol. 2014;2(1):1009.
30. Buonamici S, Ottaviani E, Testoni N, Montefusco V, Visani G, Bonifazi F, et al. Real-time quantitation of minimal residual disease in inv(16)-positive acute myeloid leukemia may indicate risk for clinical relapse and may identify patients in a curable state. Blood. 2002;99(2):443–9.
31. Yin JA, O'Brien MA, Hills RK, Daly SB, Wheatley K, Burnett AK. Minimal residual disease monitoring by quantitative RT-PCR in core binding factor AML allows risk stratification and predicts relapse: results of the United Kingdom MRC AML-15 trial. Blood. 2012;120(14):2826–35.
32. Burmeister T, Marschalek R, Schneider B, Meyer C, Gokbuget N, Schwartz S, et al. Monitoring minimal residual disease by quantification of genomic chromosomal breakpoint sequences

in acute leukemias with MLL aberrations. Leukemia. 2006;20(3):451–7.
33. Meyer C, Burmeister T, Groger D, Tsaur G, Fechina L, Renneville A, et al. The MLL recombinome of acute leukemias in 2017. Leukemia. 2018;32(2):273–84.
34. Alonso CN, Longo PL, Gallego MS, Medina A, Felice MS. A novel AF9 breakpoint in MLL-AF9-positive acute monoblastic leukemia. Pediatr Blood Cancer. 2008;50(4):869–71.
35. Meyer C, Burmeister T, Strehl S, Schneider B, Hubert D, Zach O, et al. Spliced MLL fusions: a novel mechanism to generate functional chimeric MLL-MLLT1 transcripts in t(11;19)(q23;p13.3) leukemia. Leukemia. 2007;21(3):588–90.
36. Rubnitz JE, Behm FG, Curcio-Brint AM, Pinheiro RP, Carroll AJ, Raimondi SC, et al. Molecular analysis of t(11;19) breakpoints in childhood acute leukemias. Blood. 1996;87(11):4804–8.
37. Gore L, Ess J, Bitter MA, McGavran L, Meltesen L, Wei Q, et al. Protean clinical manifestations in children with leukemias containing MLL-AF10 fusion. Leukemia. 2000;14(12):2070–5.
38. Dreyling MH, Schrader K, Fonatsch C, Schlegelberger B, Haase D, Schoch C, et al. MLL and CALM are fused to AF10 in morphologically distinct subsets of acute leukemia with translocation t(10;11): both rearrangements are associated with a poor prognosis. Blood. 1998;91(12):4662–7.
39. Busson-Le Coniat M, Salomon-Nguyen F, Hillion J, Bernard OA, Berger R. MLL-AF1q fusion resulting from t(1;11) in acute leukemia. Leukemia. 1999;13(2):302–6.
40. Shinohara A, Ichikawa M, Ueda K, Takahashi T, Hangaishi A, Kurokawa M. A novel MLL-AF1p/Eps15 fusion variant in therapy-related acute lymphoblastic leukemia, lacking the EH-domains. Leuk Res. 2010;34(2):e62–3.
41. Balgobind BV, Raimondi SC, Harbott J, Zimmermann M, Alonzo TA, Auvrignon A, et al. Novel prognostic subgroups in childhood 11q23/MLL-rearranged acute myeloid leukemia: results of an international retrospective study. Blood. 2009;114(12):2489–96.
42. Cilloni D, Renneville A, Hermitte F, Hills RK, Daly S, Jovanovic JV, et al. Real-time quantitative polymerase chain reaction detection of minimal residual disease by standardized WT1 assay to enhance risk stratification in acute myeloid leukemia: a European LeukemiaNet study. J Clin Oncol. 2009;27(31):5195–201.
43. Olsson K, Gerard CJ, Zehnder J, Jones C, Ramanathan R, Reading C, et al. Real-time t(11;14) and t(14;18) PCR assays

provide sensitive and quantitative assessments of minimal residual disease (MRD). Leukemia. 1999;13(11):1833–42.
44. Kaminski MS, Tuck M, Estes J, Kolstad A, Ross CW, Zasadny K, et al. 131I-tositumomab therapy as initial treatment for follicular lymphoma. N Engl J Med. 2005;352(5):441–9.
45. van Dongen JJ, Langerak AW, Bruggemann M, Evans PA, Hummel M, Lavender FL, et al. Design and standardization of PCR primers and protocols for detection of clonal immunoglobulin and T-cell receptor gene recombinations in suspect lymphoproliferations: report of the BIOMED-2 concerted action BMH4-CT98-3936. Leukemia. 2003;17(12):2257–317.
46. Gruber TA, Larson Gedman A, Zhang J, Koss CS, Marada S, Ta HQ, et al. An Inv(16)(p13.3q24.3)-encoded CBFA2T3-GLIS2 fusion protein defines an aggressive subtype of pediatric acute megakaryoblastic leukemia. Cancer Cell. 2012;22(5):683–97.
47. Grimwade D, Hills RK, Moorman AV, Walker H, Chatters S, Goldstone AH, et al. Refinement of cytogenetic classification in acute myeloid leukemia: determination of prognostic significance of rare recurring chromosomal abnormalities among 5876 younger adult patients treated in the United Kingdom Medical Research Council trials. Blood. 2010;116(3):354–65.
48. Lim G, Choi JR, Kim MJ, Kim SY, Lee HJ, Suh JT, et al. Detection of t(3;5) and NPM1/MLF1 rearrangement in an elderly patient with acute myeloid leukemia: clinical and laboratory study with review of the literature. Cancer Genet Cytogenet. 2010;199(2):101–9.
49. Hollink IH, van den Heuvel-Eibrink MM, ST A-P, Pratcorona M, Abbas S, Kuipers JE, et al. NUP98/NSD1 characterizes a novel poor prognostic group in acute myeloid leukemia with a distinct HOX gene expression pattern. Blood. 2011;118(13):3645–56.
50. Shiba N, Ichikawa H, Taki T, Park MJ, Jo A, Mitani S, et al. NUP98-NSD1 gene fusion and its related gene expression signature are strongly associated with a poor prognosis in pediatric acute myeloid leukemia. Genes Chromosomes Cancer. 2013;52(7):683–93.
51. Zehentner BK, Cutler JA, Fritschle WK, Bennington RK, Wentzel C, Smading SR, et al. A minority of concurrent monoclonal lymphocytes and plasmacytic cells sharing light chains are genetically related in putative lymphoplasmacytic lymphoma. Leuk Res. 2011;35(12):1597–604.
52. Zehentner BK, de Baca ME, Wells DA, Loken MR. Intraclonal heterogeneity in concomitant monoclonal lymphocyte and

plasma cell populations: combining flow cytometric cell sorting with molecular monoclonality profiling. Clin Lymphoma Myeloma Leuk. 2013;13(2):214–7.
53. Burnworth B, Wang Z, Singleton TP, Bennington A, Fritschle W, Bennington R, et al. Clone-specific MYD88 L265P and CXCR4 mutation status can provide clinical utility in suspected Waldenstrom macroglobulinemia/lymphoplasmacytic lymphoma. Leuk Res. 2016;51:41–8.
54. Hovorkova L, Zaliova M, Venn NC, Bleckmann K, Trkova M, Potuckova E, et al. Monitoring of childhood ALL using BCR-ABL1 genomic breakpoints identifies a subgroup with CML-like biology. Blood. 2017;129(20):2771–81.
55. Jain P, Kantarjian H, Jabbour E, Kanagal-Shamanna R, Patel K, Pierce S, et al. Clinical characteristics of Philadelphia positive T-cell lymphoid leukemias-(De novo and blast phase CML). Am J Hematol. 2017;92(1):E3–4.
56. van der Velden VH, Hochhaus A, Cazzaniga G, Szczepanski T, Gabert J, van Dongen JJ. Detection of minimal residual disease in hematologic malignancies by real-time quantitative PCR: principles, approaches, and laboratory aspects. Leukemia. 2003;17(6):1013–34.
57. van der Velden VH, Willemse MJ, van der Schoot CE, Hahlen K, van Wering ER, van Dongen JJ. Immunoglobulin kappa deleting element rearrangements in precursor-B acute lymphoblastic leukemia are stable targets for detection of minimal residual disease by real-time quantitative PCR. Leukemia. 2002;16(5):928–36.
58. van der Velden VH, Wijkhuijs JM, Jacobs DC, van Wering ER, van Dongen JJ. T cell receptor gamma gene rearrangements as targets for detection of minimal residual disease in acute lymphoblastic leukemia by real-time quantitative PCR analysis. Leukemia. 2002;16(7):1372–80.
59. Beishuizen A, Verhoeven MA, van Wering ER, Hahlen K, Hooijkaas H, van Dongen JJ. Analysis of Ig and T-cell receptor genes in 40 childhood acute lymphoblastic leukemias at diagnosis and subsequent relapse: implications for the detection of minimal residual disease by polymerase chain reaction analysis. Blood. 1994;83(8):2238–47.
60. Kerst G, Kreyenberg H, Roth C, Well C, Dietz K, Coustan-Smith E, et al. Concurrent detection of minimal residual disease (MRD) in childhood acute lymphoblastic leukaemia by flow cytometry and real-time PCR. Br J Haematol. 2005;128(6):774–82.

61. Campana D. Minimal residual disease studies in acute leukemia. Am J Clin Pathol. 2004;122(Suppl):S47–57.
62. Bottcher S, Ritgen M, Pott C, Bruggemann M, Raff T, Stilgenbauer S, et al. Comparative analysis of minimal residual disease detection using four-color flow cytometry, consensus IgH-PCR, and quantitative IgH PCR in CLL after allogeneic and autologous stem cell transplantation. Leukemia. 2004;18(10):1637–45.
63. Malec M, van der Velden VH, Bjorklund E, Wijkhuijs JM, Soderhall S, Mazur J, et al. Analysis of minimal residual disease in childhood acute lymphoblastic leukemia: comparison between RQ-PCR analysis of Ig/TcR gene rearrangements and multicolor flow cytometric immunophenotyping. Leukemia. 2004;18(10):1630–6.
64. Sausville JE, Salloum RG, Sorbara L, Kingma DW, Raffeld M, Kreitman RJ, et al. Minimal residual disease detection in hairy cell leukemia. Comparison of flow cytometric immunophenotyping with clonal analysis using consensus primer polymerase chain reaction for the heavy chain gene. Am J Clin Pathol. 2003;119(2):213–7.
65. Zehentner BK, Fritschle W, Stelzer T, Ghirardelli KM, Hunter K, Wentzel C, et al. Minimal disease detection and confirmation in hematologic malignancies: combining cell sorting with clonality profiling. Clin Chem. 2006;52(3):430–7.
66. Bruggemann M, Droese J, Bolz I, Luth P, Pott C, von Neuhoff N, et al. Improved assessment of minimal residual disease in B cell malignancies using fluorogenic consensus probes for real-time quantitative PCR. Leukemia. 2000;14(8):1419–25.
67. Donovan JW, Ladetto M, Zou G, Neuberg D, Poor C, Bowers D, et al. Immunoglobulin heavy-chain consensus probes for real-time PCR quantification of residual disease in acute lymphoblastic leukemia. Blood. 2000;95(8):2651–8.
68. Verhagen OJ, Willemse MJ, Breunis WB, Wijkhuijs AJ, Jacobs DC, Joosten SA, et al. Application of germline IGH probes in real-time quantitative PCR for the detection of minimal residual disease in acute lymphoblastic leukemia. Leukemia. 2000;14(8):1426–35.
69. van der Velden VH, Cazzaniga G, Schrauder A, Hancock J, Bader P, Panzer-Grumayer ER, et al. Analysis of minimal residual disease by Ig/TCR gene rearrangements: guidelines for interpretation of real-time quantitative PCR data. Leukemia. 2007;21(4):604–11.
70. Terstappen LW, Loken MR. Myeloid cell differentiation in normal bone marrow and acute myeloid leukemia assessed by multidimensional flow cytometry. Anal Cell Pathol. 1990;2(4):229–40.

71. Terstappen LW, Konemann S, Safford M, Loken MR, Zurlutter K, Buchner T, et al. Flow cytometric characterization of acute myeloid leukemia. Part 1. Significance of light scattering properties. Leukemia. 1991;5(4):315–21.
72. Zeijlemaker W, Gratama JW, Schuurhuis GJ. Tumor heterogeneity makes AML a "moving target" for detection of residual disease. Cytometry B Clin Cytom. 2014;86(1):3–14.
73. Kotrova M, Trka J, Kneba M, Bruggemann M. Is next-generation sequencing the way to go for residual disease monitoring in acute lymphoblastic leukemia? Mol Diagn Ther. 2017;21(5):481–92.
74. Shlush LI, Zandi S, Mitchell A, Chen WC, Brandwein JM, Gupta V, et al. Identification of pre-leukaemic haematopoietic stem cells in acute leukaemia. Nature. 2014;506(7488):328–33.
75. Jan M, Snyder TM, Corces-Zimmerman MR, Vyas P, Weissman IL, Quake SR, et al. Clonal evolution of preleukemic hematopoietic stem cells precedes human acute myeloid leukemia. Sci Transl Med. 2012;4(149):149ra18.
76. Corces-Zimmerman MR, Hong WJ, Weissman IL, Medeiros BC, Majeti R. Preleukemic mutations in human acute myeloid leukemia affect epigenetic regulators and persist in remission. Proc Natl Acad Sci U S A. 2014;111(7):2548–53.
77. Steensma DP, Bejar R, Jaiswal S, Lindsley RC, Sekeres MA, Hasserjian RP, et al. Clonal hematopoiesis of indeterminate potential and its distinction from myelodysplastic syndromes. Blood. 2015;126(1):9–16.
78. Young AL, Wong TN, Hughes AE, Heath SE, Ley TJ, Link DC, et al. Quantifying ultra-rare pre-leukemic clones via targeted error-corrected sequencing. Leukemia. 2015;29(7):1608–11.
79. van Dongen JJ, van der Velden VH, Bruggemann M, Orfao A. Minimal residual disease diagnostics in acute lymphoblastic leukemia: need for sensitive, fast, and standardized technologies. Blood. 2015;125(26):3996–4009.
80. Langerak AW, Bruggemann M, Davi F, Darzentas N, van Dongen JJM, Gonzalez D, et al. High-throughput Immunogenetics for clinical and research applications in immunohematology: potential and challenges. J Immunol. 2017;198(10):3765–74.
81. Ladetto M, Bruggemann M, Monitillo L, Ferrero S, Pepin F, Drandi D, et al. Next-generation sequencing and real-time quantitative PCR for minimal residual disease detection in B-cell disorders. Leukemia. 2014;28(6):1299–307.
82. Bolouri H, Farrar JE, Triche T Jr, Ries RE, Lim EL, Alonzo TA, et al. The molecular landscape of pediatric acute myeloid leukemia reveals recurrent structural alterations and age-specific mutational interactions. Nat Med. 2018;24(1):103–12.

Chapter 4
Monitoring AML Response Using "Difference from Normal" Flow Cytometry

Michael R. Loken, Lisa Eidenschink Brodersen, and Denise A. Wells

Introduction

Flow cytometry can be used to monitor response to therapy by discriminating between normal regenerating hematopoietic cells in the bone marrow and any remaining acute myeloid leukemia (AML) which abnormally expresses cell surface antigens [1]. Maturing normal hematopoietic cells exhibit cellular antigens (gene products) in a predictable manner as they mature from hematopoietic stem cell to the mature blood [2–4]. The gold standard approach for detecting residual AML, termed "difference from normal" (ΔN) is based on correlating the *quantitative* expression of multiple cell surface antigens (gene products) in the specimens using standardized antibody panels. The ΔN approach identifies all the normal regenerating cells within the specimen first, subtracts them away, and then detects clusters of abnormal cells within the remaining data set. Using this technique, it is

---

M. R. Loken (✉) · L. E. Brodersen · D. A. Wells
Hematologics, Inc., Seattle, WA, USA
e-mail: mrloken@hematologics.com

© Springer International Publishing AG, part of Springer Nature 2019
T. E. Druley (ed.), *Minimal Residual Disease Testing*,
https://doi.org/10.1007/978-3-319-94827-0_4

possible to define the precise composition of the specimen, identifying cells of all lineages and maturational stages as well as assessing specimen quality in addition to detecting and quantifying any abnormal cell population.

The discrimination between normal and abnormal early myeloid cells requires a precise understanding of the gene product expression on developing bone marrow cells during normal hematopoiesis [5, 6]. The exact location in flow cytometric multidimensional data space of each lineage present in bone marrow and all their maturational stages from hematopoietic stem cell (HSC) to mature blood cell can be determined [5, 6]. The accumulation of genetic abnormalities that are the basis of neoplastic transformation causes a dysregulation of the expression of the gene products resulting in cells that exhibit aberrant antigen expression [7, 8]. These abnormalities are the hallmark of the neoplastic cells and can be used to distinguish between normal regenerating bone marrow cells and aberrant hematopoietic cells [9, 10]. These abnormal cells can be found in acute myeloid leukemia (AML), myeloid blast crisis of chronic myelogenous leukemia (CML), myelodysplastic syndromes (MDS), myeloproliferative neoplasms (MPN), and other neoplastic processes [11].

This approach is 180° different from the commonly used "leukemia-associated immunophenotype" (LAIP) technique which searches for the diagnostic leukemia phenotype in the post-therapy bone marrow specimen [12, 13]. The LAIP approach focuses on the leukemia without regard to the underlying regenerative normal cell populations. Unlike LAIP, the ΔN technique does not require access to the diagnostic specimen (although knowing the detailed diagnostic phenotype is highly recommended to improve detection confidence) [14]. However, access to the diagnostic specimen is not always available, especially for reference laboratories. In addition, ΔN is unaffected by phenotypic changes that occur following chemotherapy, which are observed in patients monitored throughout their course of treatment [14, 15].

The detection of abnormal myeloid progenitor cells in this chapter was performed in a CAP/CLIA licensed clinical laboratory, not a research laboratory, with multiple technologists processing the specimens. The assay has evolved slowly over 23 years, first being applied to detect AML relapse post-hematopoietic stem cell transplant (HSCT) at the Fred Hutchinson Cancer Research Center (FHCRC) in a setting where the diagnostic phenotype of the leukemia was not available [11]. This assay requires a highly focused quality control program maximizing system stability including instrumentation, reagents, processing, and data analysis. In addition to being used clinically at the FHCRC since 1995, the assay has been validated to monitor response to therapy in AML in 3 separate clinical studies monitoring the treatment of >2000 patients. As a result of these studies, the Children's Oncology Group (COG) has proposed a change in its definition of clinical remission from a morphologic assessment of bone marrow aspirates to a flow cytometric-based analysis in order to better define risk categories [16]. The acronym, MRD, used to describe these techniques most accurately refers to "measureable residual disease" rather than "minimal residual disease" with the connotation of how the assay was performed as well as the characteristics of specificity and sensitivity used to detect the remaining leukemia as summarized in this chapter [17].

Definition of Normal

The basis of ΔN is predicated on knowing the quantitative gene product expression of each maturational stage of each lineage ($N = 12$) within stressed bone marrow specimens following therapy. Because of the maturation observed in these specimens, discrete populations of cells that are well separated from other cells based on their unique characteristics are rare. Five reference populations, however, can be routinely identified in regenerating bone marrow: mature lymphocytes, mature monocytes, mature neutrophils, promyelocytes, and uncommitted progenitor cells [18–20]. The precision of quantitative gene product expression on these 5 reference cell populations was determined from 77 randomly selected specimens obtained 1 month following chemotherapy using an analytical tool called support vector machines (SVM) in order to eliminate potential gating bias [20]. Twenty-seven of these specimens were used to train the SVMs which were then used to assess the variability of reference populations within the remaining 50 bone marrow specimens [18–20]. The assay uses 16 different cell surface markers in 9 tubes (Table 4.1). Four color combinations of monoclonal antibodies using natural fluorochromes along with two optimized light scatter properties result in an analysis in six-dimensional data space. Assessment of these data requires a multidimensional gating approach maintaining the spatial relationships between all parameters. (This is distinctly different from multiparameter flow cytometry which simply refers to collecting multiple characteristics simultaneously.) Two antibodies are replicated in each tube (CD45 and CD34) to provide a means to link data between tubes.

The quantitative expression of CD45 on the mature lymphocytes is amazingly consistent from individual to individual (Fig. 4.1) [18, 21]. These data were collected over a period of 3.5 years using three different cross-standardized flow cytometers and multiple lots of reagents in a routine clinical laboratory setting. The histogram of CD45 expression (Fig. 4.1, insert) demonstrates that gene product variability is very low *within* an individual, with 1 SD average of 0.113 log units. Eight replicates of CD45 intensity showed essentially no variation (1SD = 0.018 log units). The variability of the means of CD45 expression *between* individuals (1 SD = 0.0825 log units) is less than the variability *within* individuals. These data suggest that the amount of CD45 expressed on mature lymphocytes from individual to individual is a biologic constant, independent of time, instrument, reagent lot, technician, chemotherapy, or HSCT.

Similar data can be obtained for CD34 expression on the uncommitted progenitor cells [18]. The standard deviation of

TABLE 4.1 Monoclonal antibody combinations

Tube	Monoclonal antibodies			
	FITC	PE	PERCP	APC
1	Autofluorescence	Autofluorescence	CD45	CD34
Clone			*2D1 (BD)*	
2	HLA-DR	CD11b	CD45	CD34
Clone	*L243 (BD)*	*D12 (BD)*		
3	CD36	CD38	CD45	CD34
Clone	*FA6.152(BC)*	*HB7(BD)*		
4	CD16	CD13	CD45	CD34
Clone	*3G8(BD)*	*L138 (BD)*		
5	CD14	CD33	CD45	CD34
Clone	*MΦ/P9(BD)*	*P67.6(BD)*		
6	CD7	CD56	CD45	CD34
Clone	*4H9(BD)*	*My31(BD)*		
7	CD38	CD117	CD45	CD34
Clone	*HIT2(in vitro)*	*104D2(BD)*		
8	CD36	CD64	CD45	CD34
Clone	*FA6.152(BC)*	*22(T)*		
9	CD19	CD123	CD45	CD34
Clone	*4G7(BD)*	*9F5(BD)*		

BD: BD Biosciences, San Jose, CA, USA
BC: Beckman Coulter, Brea, CA, USA
Invitro: Invitrogen™, Thermo Fisher Scientific, San Diego, CA, USA
Trillium Diagnostics, LLC, Brewer, ME, USA

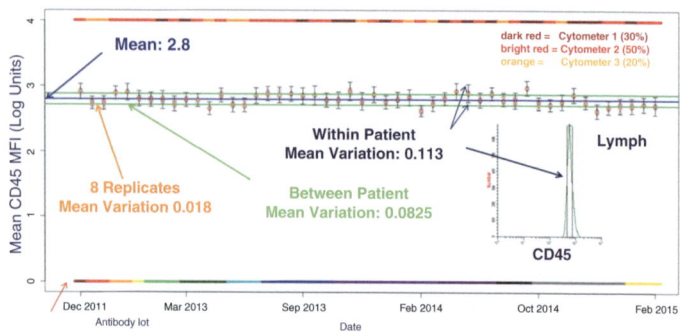

Figure 4.1 CD45 intensity variation (CD45-PerCP) on mature lymphocytes for 50 randomly selected pediatric bone marrow specimens. The top colors identify the instrument used for analysis. The bottom colors reflect the lot of antibodies used for staining. The average standard deviation (SD) of the CD45 histogram (within patient variation, insert, whiskers) was 0.113 log units. Replicate staining (CD45 is repeated eight times for each patient) showed an average SD of 0.018 log units, while the variation of the mean intensity between individuals was 0.0825 log units, green lines

CD34 intensity *within* individuals averages 0.152 log units, slightly broader than CD45 expression on the mature lymphocytes (Fig. 4.2, *insert*). Eight replicates of CD34 show a variability of 0.0167 log units. The variability of the mean intensity of CD34 *between* individuals is almost 1/3 of the variation *within* an individual (0.0638 log units). Again this suggests that the variability of amount of CD34 expressed on the uncommitted progenitor cells *within* an individual is almost three times greater than the variability of the means *between* individuals. In other words, the amount of CD34 expressed on uncommitted progenitor cells is also a biologic constant.

The quantitative expression of these gene products is independent of age [19]. The amount of CD34 expressed on adult patients recovering from treatment for AML is the same as seen in pediatric patients, Fig. 4.3. The constancy of gene product expression in both pediatric and adult individuals has been demonstrated for CD7, CD11b, CD13, CD14, CD16,

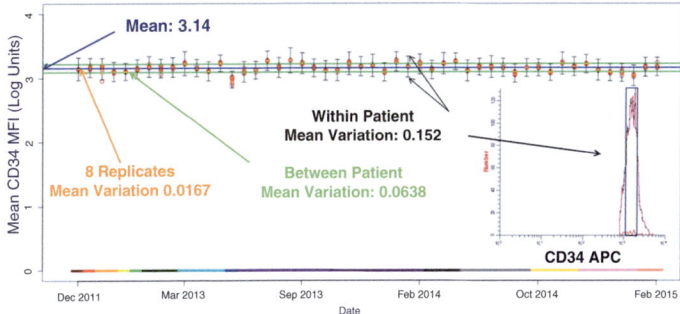

FIGURE 4.2 Variation of CD34intensities (CD34 APC) for the uncommitted progenitor cells, expressing high levels of CD34 and CD33 in the same 50 randomly selected pediatric bone marrow specimens studied in Fig. 4.1 [18]. Different lots of reagents are depicted at the bottom. The average SD for the CD34 histograms within a patient was 0.152 log units. Replicate staining averaged 0.0167 log units (1SD), while the variation of the means of CD34 from individual to individual was only 0.0638 (1SD)

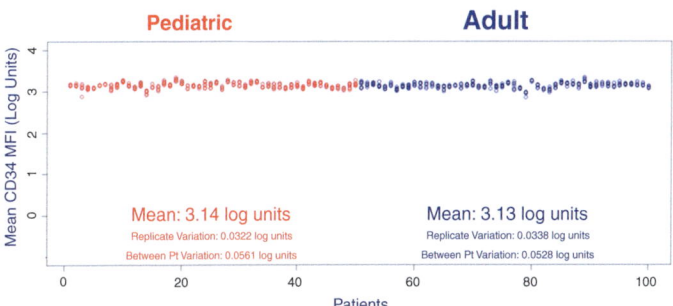

FIGURE 4.3 Comparison of intensities of CD34 expression on the uncommitted progenitor cells for 50 pediatric and adult patients on normal bone marrow cells following treatment for AML [19]

CD19, CD34, CD36, CD45, CD56, CD64, and CD123 [18, 19]. Two gene products that are related to cell activation, CD38 and HLA-DR, were highly variable and did not follow this pattern. The one gene product identified that showed higher variability between individuals than within individuals was CD33 [18, 19]. Recent studies have shown that there are genetic polymorphisms at the single-nucleotide level (SNP) that regulate the expression of amount of CD33 [22].

The assay stability has been demonstrated for 13 years extending from COG AAML03P1 and AAML0531 to AAML1031 as well as to adults treated for AML (Figs. 4.4 and 4.5). These data show that the expression of gene products on

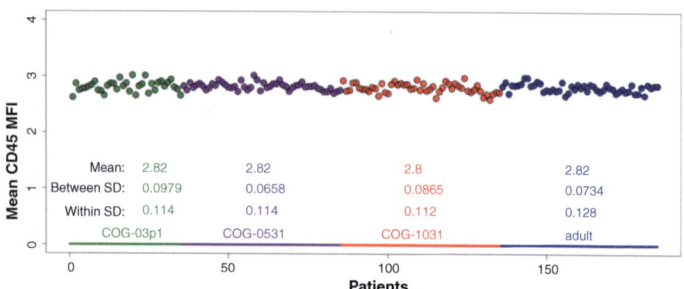

FIGURE 4.4 Comparison of CD45 intensity on lymphocytes from randomly selected patients for three separate AML clinical studies and adult patients treated for AML. The data were collected for COG AAML03p1 from February 2004 to February 2006, for AAML0531 from August 2006 to March 2010, and AAML1031 from December 2011 to February 2015. The collection of data for the adult group overlapped with AAML1031

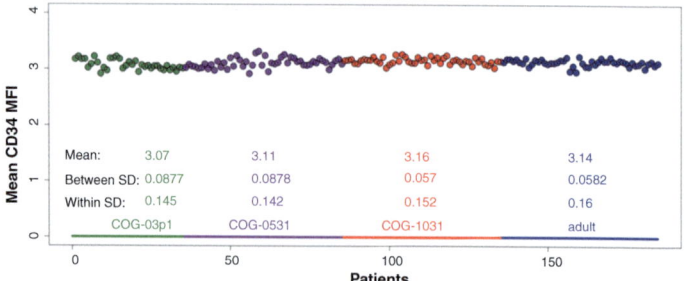

FIGURE 4.5 Intensity of expression of CD34 on uncommitted progenitor cells for randomly selected patients from the three clinical trials and adult patients described in Fig. 4.4

normal bone marrow specimens from patients treated for AML has been constant over this time period, independent of instrument, reagent lots, processing technologist, age of the individual (infant to 74 years old), stress within the bone marrow (all are post-chemotherapy), or even HSCT.

The stability of the analytic process was extended to light scatter, especially right angle or side scatter (SSC) as a measure of cellular granularity. The relationship of CD45/SSC is an important factor in identifying cells of different lineages and maturational stages within bone marrow, Fig. 4.6 [18]. Normalization of these parameters to constant position for lymphocytes demonstrates the consistent relationships between these analytical parameters for the reference populations from the 50 patients even

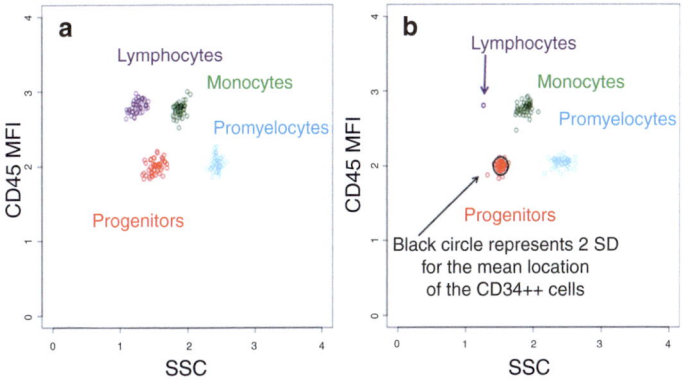

FIGURE 4.6 CD45/log SSC relationships for reference populations for 50 randomly selected pediatric bone marrow specimens (see Fig. 4.1). (**a**) The CD45 vs. SSC position of mature lymphocytes (purple), uncommitted progenitor cells (red), mature monocytes (green), and promyelocytes (blue). (**b**) Normalization of the position of the reference populations to lymphocytes. The lymphocytes (purple) were moved to the same location, and the corresponding positions of the other reference parameters were translocated using the same vector for each patient. The solid oval represents the variation of the normalized position of the uncommitted progenitor cells in the CD45 dimension (± 2 SD, y-axis) and the SSC dimension (± 2 SD, x-axis)

though the data were collected on 3 different, yet cross-calibrated, flow cytometers.

Mutations Affect Phenotypic Expression

Analysis of the flow cytometric data requires a detailed understanding of the changes in gene product expression during development from HSC to mature blood cells for each of the lineages found in bone marrow. The process of cellular maturation is not continuous but proceeds in a stepwise manner, in which multiple cellular processes change simultaneously [6, 21]. The phenotypic and cellular changes that occur at the same time of development require coordination, including turning on or off genes, up- or downregulation of amounts of gene products, gene splicing, and control of DNA synthesis [21]. The maturation of cells can then be divided into distinct stages which, for the neutrophils, match those stages identified by changes in morphology [2–5]. This precise timing, quantitative expression, RNA splicing, and DNA synthesis require a level of coordination of diverse cellular processes that is more complex than previously recognized. It is this coordination and regulation of gene products that is disrupted during leukemogenesis by the various mutational events resulting in neoplastic transformation. We now know multiple combinations of genetic abnormalities result in phenotypic changes that are unique for each leukemia [8]. This explains early studies showing that leukemia phenotypes are not only different from their normal counterparts but that each leukemia displays a unique phenotype [7,8,23]. Leukemia at presentation may consist of multiple clones that exist in different proportions and may have differential sensitivity to chemotherapy. Therapy can eliminate the sensitive clones leaving resistant clones leading to relapse with a change in phenotype. In addition, essentially all AML phenotypes exhibit maturational heterogeneity as well. Therefore, it is not unexpected that phenotypic changes reflecting these additional clones often occur following chemotherapy when comparing the diagnostic and relapse phenotypes [14].

The phenotypic abnormalities observed in AML include lineage infidelity (expression of lymphoid antigens such as CD7, CD19, CD56), antigenic asynchrony (immature antigens expressed on mature cells or quantitative differences between multiple antigens), antigenic absence (lack of expression of normal myeloid antigens such as CD13 or CD33), and quantitative expression differences, (over- or underexpression of gene products) [8]. The ΔN approach can identify all of these types of abnormalities, while the alternative LAIP approach is often dependent on lineage infidelity and antigenic absence. Quantitative differences are difficult to assess using tandem-conjugated antibodies required in assays that incorporate more than four immunofluorescence probes because of fluorophore instability and noise introduced in correcting for emission spectral overlap.

Specimen Composition and Quality

The approach of ΔN focuses first on the normal cells within the specimen providing quality control of the assay for the entire process. The reference populations must reside in the exact multidimensional locations defined by the immunofluorescence markers that are observed for other normal bone marrow specimens. From the analysis of the normal reference cell populations, it is possible to assess the specimen in terms of both composition and quality. The relative proportions of each cell type can be determined, their distribution from immature to mature can be ascertained (shift to the left or right for all lineages, not just myeloid), and nonviable cells can be identified and quantified. For example, if the mature lymphocytes are identified at 70–80% of the specimen (usually these cells represent 10–20% of nucleated cells), the myeloid cells have not regenerated, and therefore the specimen is not a representative of a normal bone marrow (lymphoid predominance). If the neutrophils are predominantly mature phenotypes, the specimen is considered hemodilute since mature neutrophils should comprise only 30% of the maturing myeloid cells in a marrow specimen [24]. The assay utilizes the same specimen volume throughout; therefore, if 200 k events cannot be collected for each tube, this indicates a hypocellular marrow. The analysis of the residual normal components within a specimen provides an excellent internal control to define how the marrow aspirate compares to a normal cellular specimens. Specimen quality is reported as (1) adequate (100–200 k cells collected with minimal hemodilution and few nonviable cells), (2) suboptimal (<100 k cells collected or significant hemodilution, increased nonviable cells or EDTA anticoagulant), and (3) inadequate (low numbers of cells collected, low numbers of progenitor cells identified, significant hemodilution, lymphoid predominance, increased nonviable cells).

Once the specimen quality is assessed, abnormal cell populations within the progenitor cell or monocyte regions by CD45/log SSC are determined using the multidimensional data analysis approach [25]. This ΔN analysis does not depend on the initial phenotype but simply is based on identifying clusters of events (at least 40) that are at least 0.5 log units separated from normal cell populations.

During the analytical phase of the test, two analysts must assess each specimen independently. They then compare their findings and either agree (with certainty) to the presence of an abnormal myeloid progenitor cell population or to no evidence of residual disease. In rare instances if there is disagreement, the analysts compare their findings and come to an agreed conclusion. There must be uniformity of agreement, or the specimen is called *negative* (or in some cases suspicious) in order to reduce the possibility of false positive reports. The focus of the analysis is on *specificity*, not sensitivity.

Lower Level of Detection

The lower level of detection of the assay is set at 0.02% for specimens with 200 k cells collected for each tube. An abnormal cluster of at least 40 cells must be identified demonstrating at least 2 phenotypic abnormalities that place the cell population at least 0.5 decades away from normal hematopoietic cells. An example of lower level of detection can be visualized by diluting a diagnostic specimen into a normal bone marrow, Fig. 4.7. The abnormal cell population was identified based on low levels of CD38 on the CD34-positive population (middle dot plots) and by reduced CD33 on the CD34 bright cells (lower dot plots). This population could then be identified in the CD45/log SSC dot plots even at a dilution of 1/10,000.

A follow-up specimen from this patient was obtained 28 days after the first induction chemotherapy (Fig. 4.8). A population of abnormal cells could be detected at 0.02% at this early time point after induction exhibiting the same phenotype identified in the diagnostic specimen. A third specimen on this patient was obtained 9 months following the initial induction demonstrating relapse at 60% with the same phenotype identified in the diagnostic specimen and after the first induction course (Fig. 4.9). Together these data demonstrate the lower level of detection of the system and stability of the leukemia phenotype and analysis over time.

Performance Characteristics

Monitoring a single patient throughout the course of treatment provides an excellent demonstration of how consistent the data are over time in a case where additional subclones did not appear. The initial specimen submitted on a patient (different from the previous illustration) followed induction chemotherapy, so no diagnostic phenotype was available for comparison. A "suspicious" population was reported on that specimen at 0.01%, below the clinical cutoff, that could be identified in two separate analytic tubes, Fig. 4.10a. A second specimen was submitted 1 month later that showed 1.5% abnormal cells with the same phenotype as was identified in the previous "suspicious" specimen (Fig. 4.10b). After another 3 months of chemotherapy, a third submitted specimen was

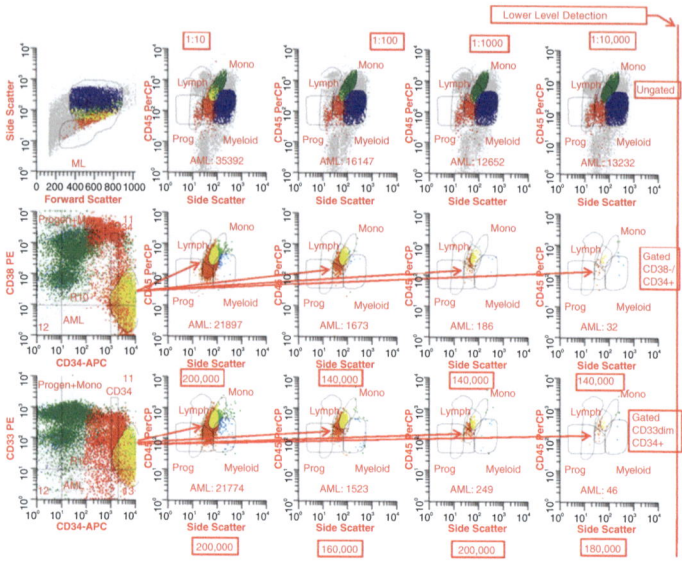

FIGURE 4.7 A diagnostic AML specimen was diluted into a normal bone marrow specimen. The leukemia population identified by CD34 and dim/negative CD38 is shown in the center plots, while the leukemia identified by dim CD33 and CD34 is shown in the bottom plots. The same population of cells could be identified in the CD45/log SSC plots even when the leukemia was diluted 1:10,000 in normal bone marrow. A cluster of events representing the leukemia can be seen at the highest dilution. The dilutions are shown in the upper boxes. The total cells counted in each specimen are shown below each dot plot

termed inadequate, low cell counts, and low viability. Two weeks later, an additional specimen was submitted without intervening chemotherapy and identified 1.6% abnormal myeloid progenitor cells with a similar phenotype to that previously identified but with a decrease in expression of HLA-DR (Fig. 4.10c). A final specimen from this patient was obtained 2 months later (7 months after the first specimen, Fig. 4.10d); however, shipment was delayed 1 week, and the specimen was collected into the wrong anticoagulant (EDTA). This last specimen was then processed 8 days after collection. Leukemia could still be identified at 0.2% with the same

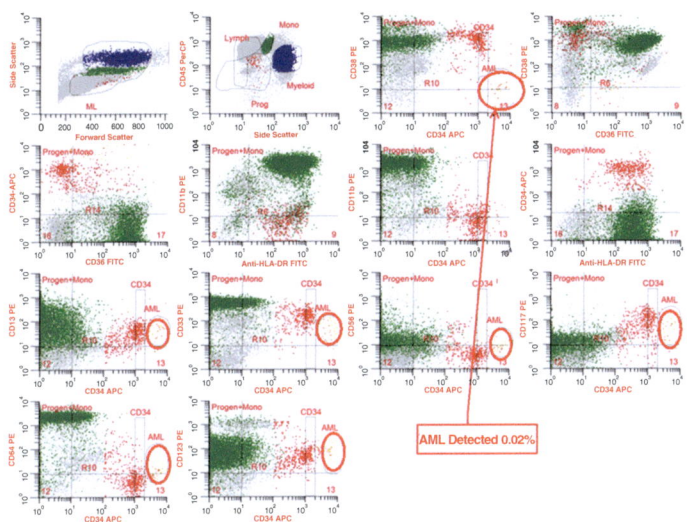

FIGURE 4.8 Analysis of the end of induction #1 (EOI#1) specimen from the same patient shown in Fig. 4.7. A distinct population of cells can be identified at 0.02% in this clinical specimen with the same phenotype identified at diagnosis

phenotypic pattern, but with a loss of HLA-DR, Fig. 4.10. These data show that some antigens are stable in fluorescence intensity spanning a 7-month period of treatment; however, others (such as HLA-DR in this case) can change.

Assay Validation

The key question to be answered in the detection of abnormal myeloid progenitor cells is: how reliable are the results based on a subjective, multidimensional assessment of the data? In other words, how *specific* is the assay? Specificity of the assay is more important than assay sensitivity although it is more difficult to ascertain. Specificity and sensitivity of the analysis are predicated on which tests are used to validate the assay. Three distinctly different methods can be used to determine whether or not the cell population identified as being

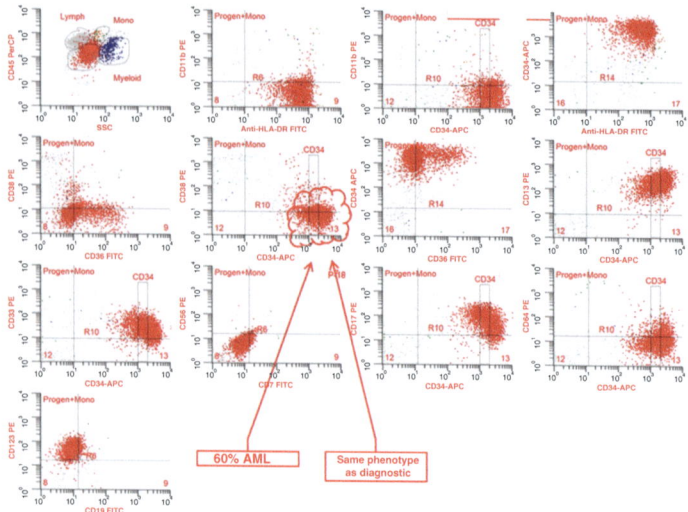

FIGURE 4.9 Analysis of a bone marrow specimen submitted 9 months following induction chemotherapy from the same patient shown in Figs. 4.7 and 4.8. The patient is now in relapse with the same phenotype observed at diagnosis

abnormal is, in fact, a neoplastic cell population: direct, correlative, and indirect.

Direct assay validation requires purification of the population identified as abnormal, followed by an independent or orthogonal means to prove that the cells identified are neoplastic. Purified cells can be assayed for *known* molecular markers or FISH abnormalities within the neoplastic cells. However, not all neoplastic processes possess an identifiable, measurable genetic marker. In addition, detection of abnormal cell populations may not have access to the diagnostic phenotype or genotype. Those neoplastic processes that do have known genetic abnormalities do not necessarily represent the totality of all neoplastic phenotypes as there is a direct relationship between genotype and phenotype [26]. Therefore, assays used to confirm neoplastic cells that focus on FISH or molecular abnormalities may not work in every

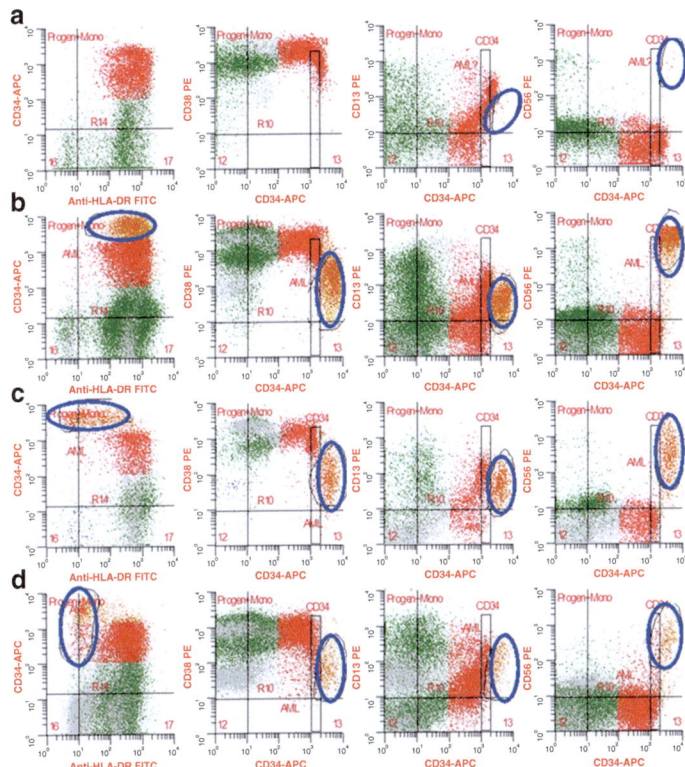

FIGURE 4.10 Monitoring a single patient over time without access to a diagnostic phenotype. (**a**) Post-induction specimen revealed a suspicious cell population at 0.01%. (**b**) One month later the abnormal population was identified at 1.5%, confirming the presence of AML in the previous specimen. (**c**) The AML was identified at 1.6% in a subsequent specimen following additional chemotherapy. (**d**) The final specimen received on this patient was collected 2 months later in the wrong anticoagulant (EDTA) and was delayed in shipping for a week. The AML was still identifiable at 0.2%

case nor be representative of all phenotypes identified as abnormal. In addition, abnormal markers identified at diagnosis may be absent following chemotherapy because of clonal selection.

One direct analytical approach to assay validation that is independent of the underlying genetic markers and is useful for all neoplastic processes is chimerism following myeloablative HSCT. Distinction between donor and recipient can be made using short tandem repeat analysis (STR), a standardized technique used in forensics and paternity cases [27]. A comparison between STR expression of the purified abnormal cells to the pre-HSCT specimen and an internal control of either purified lymphocytes or neutrophils post-HSCT can distinguish between donor and recipient origin of the cell populations. Neoplastic cells post-HSCT are necessarily recipient, while the regenerative cells will be donor origin. (The ΔN approach has been used to identify neoplastic processes arising from the donor cells [28]).

Direct confirmation is the approach used in clinical practice when patients are not enrolled on clinical study. A specimen is submitted for leukemia detection, often without a previous diagnostic specimen for comparison. Detection of low levels of abnormal cells is confirmed by cell sorting followed by FISH or molecular tests whenever possible. This approach can only be used on a subset of patients exhibiting a detectable genetic marker.

Correlative assay validation is similar to direct assay validation without the purification of the abnormal cell population. This approach requires knowledge of the molecular or genetic abnormality in the neoplastic cells of the patient so that the detection of abnormal cells can be correlated to a separate assay done on the same specimen. This approach requires that both the phenotypic detection of cells and the correlative assay have the same sensitivity. PCRmolecular tests may be more sensitive than the flow cytometric assay, while FISH tests and karyotyping may be less sensitive. Without cell sorting, it is not possible to define which cell population contains the genetic abnormality.

Indirect assay validation is the most commonly used approach to pathology tests in which a biological response is correlated to the detection of neoplastic cells. Patients are identified as being positive for a specific characteristic; then the frequency of relapse or disease progression of those patients is compared to those that are negative for the characteristic. The most commonly used analytical technique is Kaplan-Meier analysis to determine differences in clinical outcomes based on the separation of different groups of patients. This approach is complicated by relying on a biologic response as an endpoint, often separated by months or years. Indirect assay validation requires large clinical studies of identically treated and/or randomized patients to prove significance of the assay based on statistical analysis of clinical outcomes. The endpoints may be affected by therapy or other confounding contributors to patient outcomes rather than accurately measuring the performance characteristics of the assay.

Direct Validation of ΔN Post-HSCT

A recently completed clinical trial compared the detection of AML pre- and post-allogeneic HSCT by ΔN flow cytometry with molecular detection of WT-1 [29]. In this study, which enrolled 150 individuals, the diagnostic specimen was not available for comparison for either the flow cytometric or molecular analyses. Specimens were submitted pre-HSCT as well as two time points posttransplant (nominally days 42 and 100). If aberrant myeloid progenitor cells were detected posttransplant, these cells were sorted for chimerism studies comparing the results to pre-HSCT specimens. (There was no access to the donor specimen for chimerism comparison.)

In this study, detection of abnormal myeloid progenitor cells post-HSCT specimen by flow cytometry was often the first opportunity to identify and characterize the AML cells. The goal of detection of residual disease in this setting is to have sufficient confidence in the data to convince the treating

120 M. R. Loken et al.

oncologist to intervene; therefore, the emphasis must be on specificity of residual detection. Abnormal cells were detected in 21 patients post-HSCT (0.03–78%), of which 17 specimens were successfully sorted for chimerism studies.

An example of direct confirmation of leukemia post-HSCT is illustrated in Fig. 4.11. In this patient, residual disease was detected pre-HSCT at 2.2% with essentially the same phenotype detected at 0.1% in the day 42 specimen, Fig. 4.11. Two populations of CD34-positive cells (CD34+/CD56+ and CD34+/CD56-) were sorted for STR analysis and compared to the pre-HSCT specimen.

The chimerism data show that the CD34+/CD56+ population has the same STR peaks as the pre-HSCT specimen, Fig. 4.12. However, the CD34+/CD56- population of cells has a different pattern of STR peaks indicating that this population arises from the donor. A comparison between the two sorted cell populations shows the purity of the cell fractions as assayed by STR analysis. Peaks that are observed in the

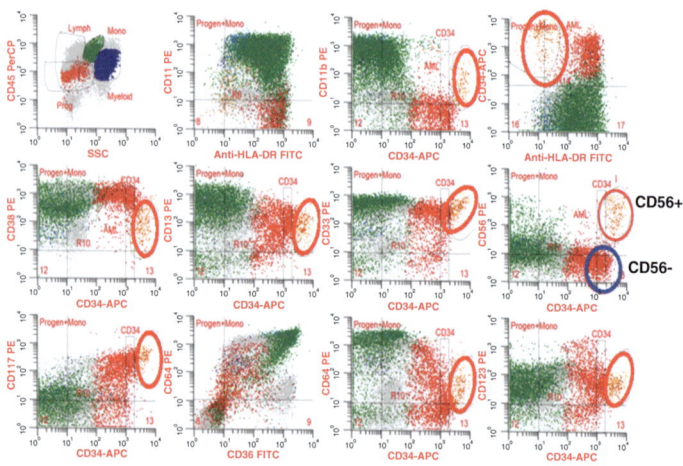

FIGURE 4.11 AML identified at 0.1% in a day 42 post-allogeneic HSCT specimen. The AML cells are identified in the red ovals. The CD34+/CD56+ and CD34 + CD56- cell populations were sorted and SCR analysis was compared to the pre-HSCT specimen; see Fig. 4.12

Chapter 4. Difference from Normal MRD 121

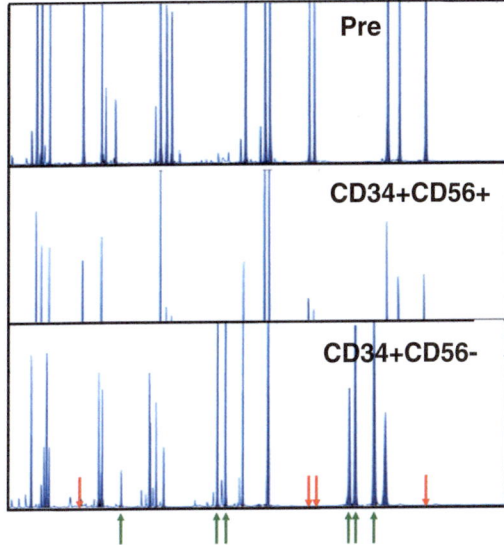

FIGURE 4.12 Comparison of STR analysis of the pre-HSCT bone marrow specimen to the sorted fractions obtained at day 42. The CD34+/CD56+ cells (Fig. 4.11) have the same peak positions as observed in the pre-HSCT specimen. The CD34+/CD56- cells exhibit different STR peaks. The green arrows indicate new peaks, while the red arrows denote peaks that are lost. The differences between the two sorted fractions are a measure of the purity of the sorted cell populations

recipient cell fractions are not identified in the donor purified cell population and vice versa. This provides an internal control that the sorted cell fractions were pure. Analysis of the day 100 specimen for this patient showed 45% AML with the same phenotype seen at day 42, demonstrating a clear relapse after 2 months.

Of the 17 patients identified to have aberrant myeloid progenitor cells post-HSCT and analyzed by chimerism analysis, 15 were confirmed to be recipient in the sorted cell population. All 15 relapsed on the study. Retrospective analysis of the two post-HSCT specimens that were not confirmed to be recipient and who did not relapse showed that one specimen was the result of a technical error. The second specimen was called suspicious based on a population of cells at 0.06%, identified at both days 42 and 100 exhibiting a *single* abnormality of high expression of CD34+ co-expressing CD7+. This suspicious population could not be confirmed by chimerism, demonstrating the importance of using an orthogonal assay to prove the origin of the abnormal cells. Without a diagnostic specimen for comparison, it is difficult to be certain about small populations of cells that do not exhibit multiple abnormal antigen features. The combination of ΔN detection of abnormal cells followed by chimerism confirmation provided 100% specificity in this study even without a diagnostic specimen for comparison.

Retrospective analysis of the pre-HSCT specimens using the relapse phenotypes as a pattern suggests that patients who relapse, but who were not identified as positive in the pretransplant specimen, exhibit phenotypes that are not similar to normal. This means that the relapse phenotype was significantly different from normal and could have been identified in the pre-HSCT specimen. In the retrospective analysis of all the pre-HSCT specimens, 1/3 did not have an "adequate" specimen quality. Patients who are poised to undergo HSCT have often received multiple courses of chemotherapy, and marrow reconstitution may be impaired. Among those relapse patients with an adequate specimen submitted pre-HSCT, only 2/9 could be called positive (both at 0.04%) in a retrospective analysis. Three additional pre-HSCT specimens were retrospectively called "suspicious" at levels below 0.08%, while the remaining four had no evidence of relapse tumor above 0.02%.

Of the ten patients originally identified as positive pre-HSCT (0.04–14%), 9/10 either relapsed or died of treatment-related mortality following transplant [29]. All of these patients were defined at the submitting institutions as in clinical remission (CR) with <5% morphologic blasts. Interestingly, flow cytometry identified four patients with more than 5% abnormal blasts suggesting that the morphologic identification of residual disease for these patients was not adequate.

Correlative Validation of Response to Therapy

The combination of multiple technologies can provide a better understanding of disease processes, increased confidence in the assays, and enhanced interpretation of results. In order to correlate the results from different technologies on unsorted specimens, the two assays must have similar characteristics for sensitivity and specificity in the detection of the abnormal population. However, interpretation of correlative results may still be ambiguous in a clinical setting (Fig. 4.13).

A bone marrow aspirate from a 13-year-old patient was submitted for residual disease detection with no other clinical information and no diagnostic phenotype for comparison. Upon analysis of the 4-day-old specimen, it was clear that there was a shift to the left demonstrated by an increase in promyelocytes (34% of myeloid cells), Fig. 4.13b. The progenitor cells (*red,* Fig. 4.13a) were phenotypically normal; however, an increase in mast cells (2.5%) was evident in the analysis, Fig. 4.13c. These mast cells were shown to be aberrant with the expression of both CD2 and CD25, Fig. 4.13d–f [30, 31]. These flow cytometric results were consistent with systemic mastocytosis with a background of normal but immature myeloid cells. Upon contacting the sending institution, the diagnostic cytogenetics showed t(8;21) allowing both molecular and FISH studies to be used to correlate the results. Molecular studies using RT-PCR for AML1(RUNX1)-ETO(RUNX1T1) was positive at 0.087 normalized copy numbers.

In order to interpret the molecular results, it was necessary to understand which cell population(s) contained the abnormal genetic marker. Cell sorting of the mast cells and the CD34-positive progenitor cells was performed for analysis by FISH, Fig. 4.13c. The mast cell fraction showed 128/200 exhibiting the translocation, while both the CD34-positive fraction and the purified CD3-positive cells (negative control) showed no evidence of this genetic abnormality.

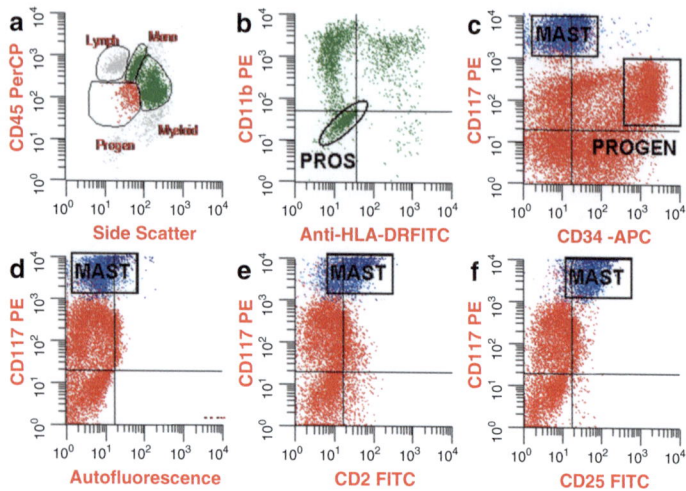

FIGURE 4.13 A bone marrow aspirate submitted for detection of residual AML. (**a**) The proportions of cells in the major lineages were within expected ranges. (**b**) An increase in the proportions of promyelocytes (34% of myeloid cells) suggested early marrow recovery posttreatment. (**c**) Mast cells were identified at 2.5% and shown to be aberrant with the expression of CD2 and CD25 (**d**–**f**). The mast cells, CD34-positive progenitor cells, and CD3-positive T cells were sorted for analysis by FISH (**c**)

This case illustrates the importance of interpretation what a positive result means for an individual patient. The genetic abnormality was confined to the mature, nondividing mast cell population not the immature progenitor cells. Similar results were observed for a patient both pre- and up to 18 months post-HSCT without relapse after 5 years [32]. Detection of abnormal cells by immunofluorescence, molecular, or genetic studies must be integrated with an understanding that identification of a genetic abnormality may not predict an adverse outcome. Assays that are validated by monitoring clinical trials may need modification or enhancement when applied to specific, unique patient situations.

Indirect Validation to Monitoring Response to Therapy

Three separate clinical trials sponsored by COG enrolling >2000 have been monitored using the ΔN approach to measure response to therapy. The COG clinical trial AAML0531 was a phase 3 study of the use of Mylotarg® (gemtuzumab ozogamicin, humanized CD33 coupled to calicheamicin; Pfizer, Inc.) as an upfront drug in the treatment of AML in pediatric patients [33]. Mylotarg is the first antibody/drug conjugate to be used as a targeted therapy for cancer patient [34]. Patients were randomized to different arms with half receiving the new drug, Fig. 4.14.

Flow cytometry using the ΔN approach was performed by Hematologics at diagnosis (in most but not all cases) and then after each course of chemotherapy, end of the first induction (EOI#1), end of the second induction (EOI#2), and after consolidation. Addition specimens were obtained at

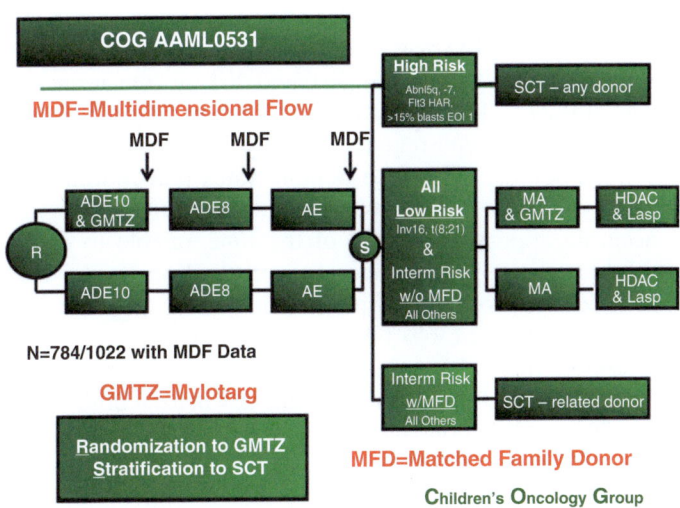

FIGURE 4.14 Clinical scheme for treatment of patients on AAML0531 [33]

later stages of therapy for many but not all patients. Detection of "complete response" (CR) in this study was performed by the standard morphologic assessment of bone marrow aspirates counting the proportion of blasts at the treating institution. One hundred eighty-five patients (24%) failed to achieve CR with 94 partial remissions (PR, 5–15% blasts) and 91 with persistent disease (PD, >15% blasts, defined as a high-risk group in this study) [35].

Of the 24% who did not achieve CR by morphology, 1/3 of the patients demonstrated normal phenotype on the myeloid progenitor cells by flow cytometry, i.e., no evidence of disease. Those patients that had >5% morphologic blasts but were negative by flow cytometry had standard outcome not poor outcome, Fig. 4.15. The outcomes for the MRD-negative patients were the same whether or not the morphologist counted <5% morphologic blasts. Of those patients with PD and >15% blasts ($N = 91$), 25 patients were called negative by flow cytometry with outcomes no different from patients with <5% morphologic blasts and no evidence of disease by flow cytometry. In the previous AML study (AAML03p1 where all patients received Mylotarg), a similar group of six patients were classified as PD by morphology but were phenotypically normal. All six patients were alive and disease-free at the end of the study [9]. Together these results show that high levels of normal phenotype regenerating myeloid progenitor cells are not poor risk. This also demonstrates that morphology using a cutoff of 5% or even 15% when counting blasts is inaccurate approximately 1/3 of the time, unable to distinguish between normal regenerating myeloid progenitor cells and residual leukemia. Morphology is neither sensitive (5% cutoff) nor specific (36% false positive cases).

Residual disease was detected at the end of induction #1 (see Fig. 4.14) by flow cytometry using ΔN in 31% of the cases ($N = 784$) and demonstrated a significant difference in outcome, Fig. 4.16. Interestingly, the level of residual disease detection at this early time point was independent of outcome, Fig. 4.17. The disease-free survival of patients with >5% residual disease (easy to identify by flow cytometry) and

Chapter 4. Difference from Normal MRD 127

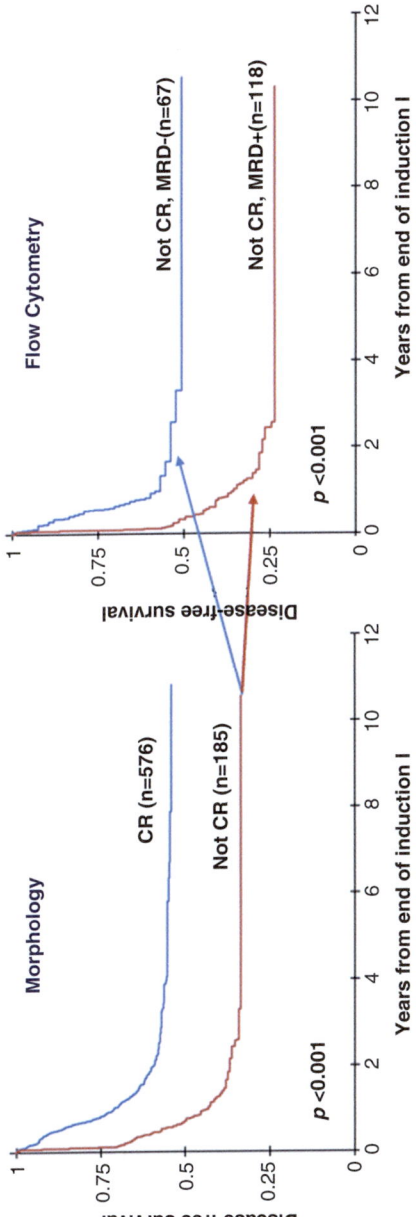

FIGURE 4.15 *Left*: Disease-free survival for patients classified as morphologic No CR. *Right*: Disease-free survival of the No CR patients stratified by phenotyping the myeloid progenitor cells. The MRD- patients exhibited increased progenitor cells, but these were normal phenotype. Their survival was not different from MDF- patients who had <5% morphologic blasts [35]

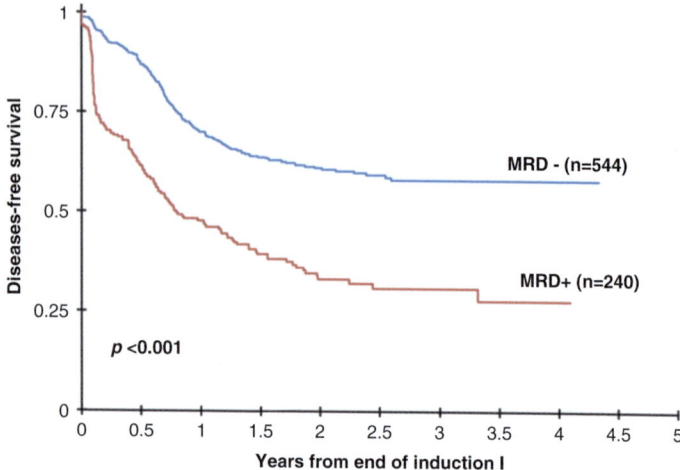

FIGURE 4.16 Survival of patients identified as harboring residual disease based on flow cytometry. 31% of all patients were classified as MRD+ with a disease-free survival of 28% as compared to the MRD- group with a survival of 60% [36]

those identified as having 0.02–0.1% (difficult) was the same. Patients with 0.1–1% as well as patients with 1–5% also showed the same survival. The difference in these curves was the kinetics of relapse; those with lower levels of leukemia took longer to relapse. The similarity of survival between patients with high levels of leukemia and low levels of leukemia demonstrate that the *specificity* in detecting residual disease is the same at both the high- and low-detection limits. This means that although the identification of low levels of leukemia is difficult, in this blinded study, few if any false positive patients were included.

Similar correlations with outcome were identified in patients after the second round of chemotherapy, Fig. 4.18. Patients who were positive in specimens collected at EOI#1 and who were also positive at EOI#2 showed a 25% disease-free survival (purple). Patients who cleared their disease going from MRD+ at EOI#1 to MRD- after EOI#2 (red) showed a slightly better outcome but was still very poor

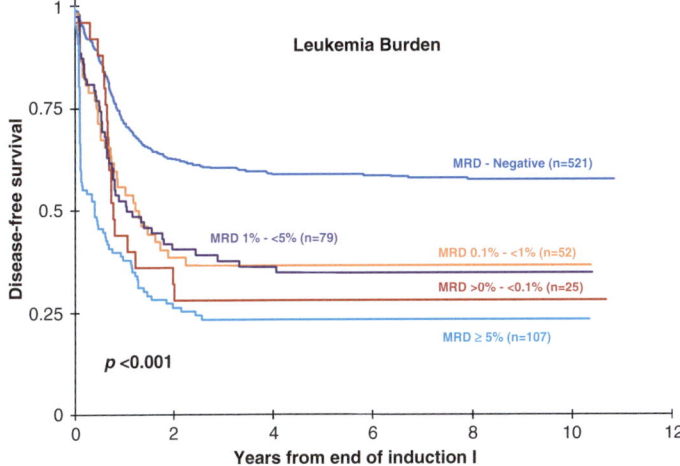

FIGURE 4.17 Survival curves for patients with varying levels of MRD identified at the end of induction #1. The disease-free survival was the same whether the patient had >5% leukemic blasts or <0.1% leukemic blasts. These data show that the specificity at the high and low ranges of the assay is the same. The difference between these patient groups was the kinetics of relapse; those patients with lower leukemia burden took longer to relapse [36, 37]

compared to patients who had no detectable residual disease at either EOI#1 or EOI#2 (blue). A small but interesting group of patients did not have detectable residual disease after the first round of chemotherapy (MRD- at EOI#1) but were positive at EOI#2 also had dismal outcomes (green). Retrospective analysis of these 12 patients revealed that the specimen quality for these patients at EOI#1 was poor. Therefore, detection of residual disease in these patients was affected by inadequate specimens. These results were the impetus to include specimen quality in the residual disease reports. It is clear that the detection of residual disease in a poor specimen is compromised.

A smaller pilot study (AAML03P1) preceded the phase 3 Mylotarg clinical trial [9, 16]. In that study, 220 patients were stratified based on residual disease detection by flow

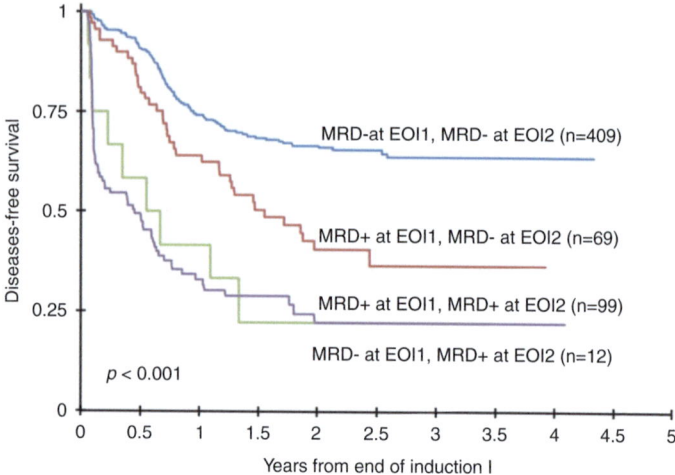

FIGURE 4.18 Residual disease measured at two different time points during therapy. Patients who were positive at both EOI1 and EOI2 (purple) as well as patients who were MRD- in the first specimen but who were detected as positive at the EOI2 (green) have the same disease-free survival. Patients who cleared their disease, MRD+ at EOI1 but MRD- at EOI2 (red), are still at high risk with a lower disease-free survival as compared to patients who showed no evidence of disease at either time point (MRD- at EOI1, MRD- at EOI2, blue)

cytometry. The 27% of patients harboring residual disease by flow cytometry had significantly worse outcomes as compared to those patients without detectable residual disease. Flow cytometry subdivided the patients who were called non-CR by morphology, identifying patients who had increased blasts but which were phenotypically normal. A small group of patients ($N = 6$) classified as persistent disease by morphology had normal phenotypes, and none of these relapsed or died.

MRD by Flow Cytometry Incorporated into Risk Stratification

In both of the AAML03P1and AAML0531 clinical studies, residual disease detection was a biological study, without using the results for treatment decisions. The incorporation of flow cytometry as a significant contribution to risk stratification along with cytogenetic and molecular results was recently presented at the American Society of Hematology (ASH) [16]. Karyotyping, immunophenotyping, molecular analysis, and next-generation sequencing were correlated to outcome for patients treated on AAML0531. Risk stratification in the AAML03P1 study utilizing limited cytogenetic and molecular groups resulted in almost 60% of patients who were deemed standard risk (Fig. 4.19a. By incorporating additional molecular and genetic markers, more patients could be categorized into high- or low-risk groups leaving 1/3 of patients classified as standard risk (Fig. 4.19b. High-risk group constituted 34% of all AML patients with an event-free survival of 26.3%. Patients with core-binding factor (CBF) AML, NPM, or CEBPA mutations constitute 33% of AML cases. The standard risk group (33%) lacking molecular or karyotypic features could be stratified based on the detection of residual disease by ΔN flow cytometry resulting in two distinct groups of patients, high risk and low risk (Fig. 4.19c). This clinical trial group has now effectively changed the definition of CR from a morphologic-based assay to flow cytometry using ΔN.

Two subsequent clinical studies (AAML1031 and AAML1531) have incorporated detection of residual disease following initial induction chemotherapy to change subsequent therapy [38]. In AAML1031 patients harboring >0.1% abnormal myeloid progenitor cells without other risk factors

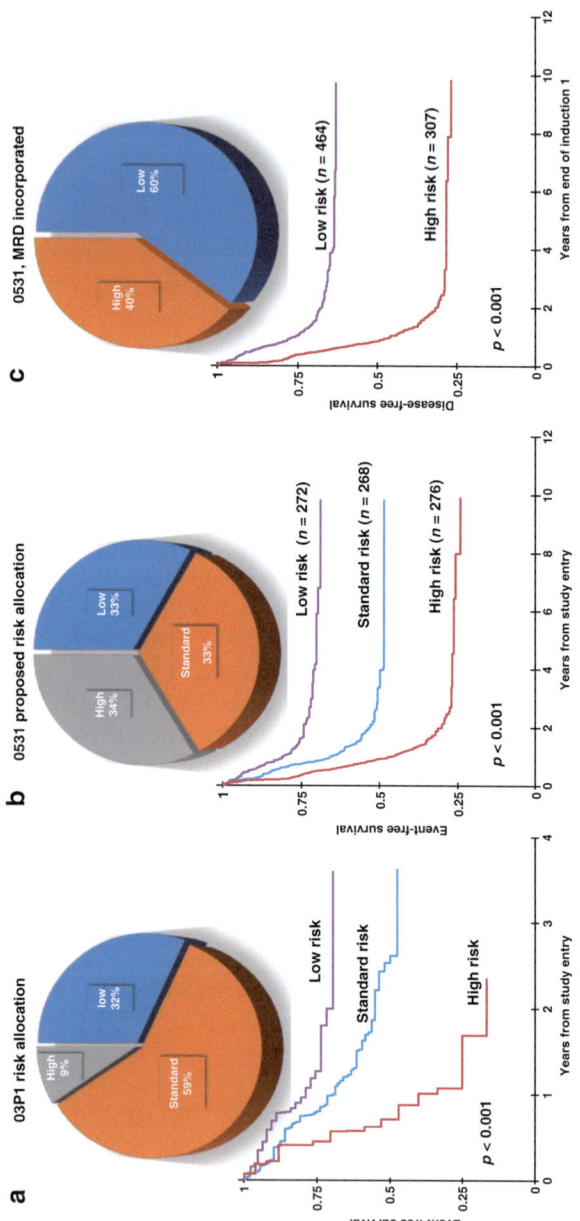

FIGURE 4.19 Proposed risk stratification for AML patients incorporating residual disease detection for patients lacking molecular or cytogenetic risk features (Standard Risk) [16]

received a more intensive chemotherapy regimen and were scheduled for an HSCT with the best available donor. In AAML1531, designed for treatment of AML of Down syndrome, patients without detectable abnormal myeloid progenitor cells receive a less intense chemotherapeutic protocol.

Acknowledgments The authors wish to thank the collaborative contributions of many individuals and groups including Soheil Meshinchi, MD, PhD; members, staff, as well as families of the Children's Oncology Group; David Jacobsohn, MD, PhD; Center for International Blood and Marrow Transplant Research; and the staff of Hematologics, Inc.

References

1. Schuurhuis GJ, Heuser M, Freeman S, Bene MC, Buccisano F, Cloos J, et al. Minimal/measurable residual disease in AML: a consensus document from the European LeukemiaNet MRD working party. Blood. 2018;131(12):1275–91.
2. Terstappen LW, Segers-Nolten I, Safford M, Shah VO, Loken MR. Monomyeloid cell differentiation in normal bone marrow assessed by multidimensional flow cytometry. In: Burger MO G, Vooijs GP, editors. Advances in analytical cellular pathology: proceedings of the first conference of the European society for analytical cellular pathology. Amsterdam: Excerpta Medica; 1990. p. 211–2.
3. Terstappen LW, Safford M, Loken MR. Flow cytometric analysis of human bone marrow. III. Neutrophil maturation. Leukemia. 1990;4(9):657–63.
4. Terstappen LW, Hollander Z, Meiners H, Loken MR. Quantitative comparison of myeloid antigens on five lineages of mature peripheral blood cells. J Leukoc Biol. 1990;48(2):138–48.
5. Loken MR, Terstappen LW, Civin CI, Fackler MJ. Flow cytometric characterization of erythroid, lymphoid and monomyeloid lineages in normal human bone marrow. In: Laerum OD, Bjerksnes R, editors. Flow cytometry in hematology. New York: Academic Press; 1992. p. 31–42.
6. Loken MR, Wells DA. Normal antigen expression in hematopoiesis: basis for interpreting leukemia phenotypes. In: Stewart C, Nicholson J, editors. Immunophenotyping. New York: Wiley Liss, Inc.; 2000. p. 133–60.

7. Terstappen LW, Segers-Nolten I, Shah VO, Safford M, Loken MR. Myeloid cell differentiation in normal bone marrow and acute myeloid leukemia assessed by multi-dimensional flow cytometry. Anal Cell Pathol. 1990;2(4):229–40.
8. Terstappen LW, Safford M, Konemann S, Loken MR, Zurlutter K, Buchner T, et al. Flow cytometric characterization of acute myeloid leukemia. Part II. Phenotypic heterogeneity at diagnosis. Leukemia. 1992;6(1):70–80.
9. Loken MR, Alonzo TA, Pardo L, Gerbing RB, Raimondi SC, Hirsch BA, et al. Residual disease detected by multidimensional flow cytometry signifies high relapse risk in patients with de novo acute myeloid leukemia: a report from Children's oncology group. Blood. 2012;120(8):1581–8.
10. Wormann B, Safford M, Konemann S, Zurlutter K, Piechotka K, Schreiber K, et al. Detection of residual leukemia cells in AML patients in complete remission. 33rd Annual Meeting of the American Society of Hematology December 6–10; Denver, CO1991.
11. Shulman HM, Wells D, Gooley T, Myerson D, Bryant E, Loken MR. The biologic significance of rare peripheral blasts after hematopoietic cell transplantation is predicted by multidimensional flow cytometry. Am J Clin Pathol. 1999;112(4):513–23.
12. San Miguel JF, Martinez A, Macedo A, Vidriales MB, Lopez-Berges C, Gonzalez M, et al. Immunophenotyping investigation of minimal residual disease is a useful approach for predicting relapse in acute myeloid leukemia patients. Blood. 1997;90(6):2465–70.
13. Macedo A, San Miguel JF, Vidriales MB, Lopez-Berges MC, Garcia-Marcos MA, Gonzalez M, et al. Phenotypic changes in acute myeloid leukemia: implications in the detection of minimal residual disease. J Clin Pathol. 1996;49(1):15–8.
14. Loken MR. Residual disease in AML, a target that can move in more than one direction. Cytometry B Clin Cytom. 2014;86(1):15–7.
15. Zeijlemaker W, Gratama JW, Schuurhuis GJ. Tumor heterogeneity makes AML a "moving target" for detection of residual disease. Cytometry B Clin Cytom. 2014;86(1):3–14. https://doi.org/10.1002/cyto.b.21134. Epub 2013 Oct 21. Review.
16. Cooper TM, Ries RE, Alonzo TA, Gerbing RB, Loken MR, Brodersen LE, et al. Revised risk stratification criteria for children with newly diagnosed acute myeloid leukemia: a report from the Children's oncology group. Blood. 2017;130(1):407.

17. Goldman JM, Gale RP. What does MRD in leukemia really mean? Leukemia. 2014;28(5):1131.
18. Loken MR, Voigt AP, Eidenschink Brodersen L, Fritschle W, Menssen AJ, Meshinchi S, et al. Consistent quantitative gene product expression: #2. Antigen intensities on bone marrow cells are invariant between individuals. Cytometry A. 2016;89(11):987–96.
19. Loken MR, Voigt AP, Eidenschink Brodersen L, Fritschle W, Menssen AJ, Wells DA. Consistent quantitative gene product expression: #3. Invariance with age. Cytometry A. 2016;89(11):997–1000.
20. Voigt AP, Eidenschink Brodersen L, Pardo L, Meshinchi S, Loken MR. Consistent quantitative gene product expression:#1.Automated identification of regenerating bone marrow cell populations using support vector machines. Cytometry A. 2016;89(11):978–86.
21. Loken MR. The mechanics of quantized hematopoiesis. In: Emandi A, Karp JE, editors. Acute leukemia: an illustrated guide to diagnosis and treatment. New York: New York Demos Medical; 2018. p. 239–54.
22. Lamba JK, Voigt AP, Chauhan L, Shin M, Aplenc R, Eidenschink Brodersen L, et al. CD33 splicing SNP regulates expression levels of CD33 in normal regenerating monocytes in AML patients. Leuk Lymphoma. 2018;59(9):2250–3. https://doi.org/10.1080/10428194.2017.1421756. Epub 2018 Jan 10.
23. Hurwitz CA, Loken MR, Graham ML, Karp JE, Borowitz MJ, Pullen DJ, et al. Asynchronous antigen expression in B lineage acute lymphoblastic leukemia. Blood. 1988;72(1):299–307.
24. Loken MR, Chu SC, Fritschle W, Kalnoski M, Wells DA. Normalization of bone marrow aspirates for hemodilution in flow cytometric analyses. Cytometry B Clin Cytom. 2009;76(1):27–36.
25. Stelzer GT, Shults KE, Loken MR. CD45 gating for routine flow cytometric analysis of human bone marrow specimens. Ann N Y Acad Sci. 1993;677:265–80.
26. Voigt AP, Brodersen LE, Alonzo TA, Gerbing RB, Menssen AJ, Wilson ER, et al. Phenotype in combination with genotype improves outcome prediction in acute myeloid leukemia: a report from Children's oncology group protocol AAML0531. Haematologica. 2017;102(12):2058–68.
27. Tautz D. Hypervariability of simple sequences as a general source for polymorphic DNA markers. Nucleic Acids Res. 1989;17(16):6463–71.

28. Sala-Torra O, Hanna C, Loken MR, Flowers ME, Maris M, Ladne PA, et al. Evidence of donor-derived hematologic malignancies after hematopoietic stem cell transplantation. Biol Blood Marrow Transplant. 2006;12(5):511–7.
29. Jacobsohn DA, Loken MR, Fei M, Adams A, Brodersen LE, Logan BR, et al. Outcomes of measurable residual disease in pediatric acute myeloid leukemia pre- and post-hematopoietic stem cell transplant: validation of difference from normal flow cytometry with chimerism studies and Wilms tumor 1 gene expression [submitted manuscript]. Biol Blood Marrow Transplant. 2018. pii: S1083–8791(18)30322–7. doi: https://doi.org/10.1016/j.bbmt.2018.06.010. [Epub ahead of print].
30. Escribano L, Diaz-Agustin B, Nunez R, Prados A, Rodriguez R, Orfao A. Abnormal expression of CD antigens in mastocytosis. Int Arch Allergy Immunol. 2002;127(2):127–32.
31. Escribano L, Garcia Montero AC, Nunez R, Orfao A, Red Espanola de M. Flow cytometric analysis of normal and neoplastic mast cells: role in diagnosis and follow-up of mast cell disease. Immunol Allergy Clin N Am. 2006;26(3):535–47.
32. Dong ZM, Ramakrishnan A, Chauncey TR, Loken MR, Zehentner BK, Wu DY, et al. Adverse effect of residual neoplastic mast cells in systemic Mastocytosis associated with acute myeloid leukemia with T(8;21)(Q22;Q22); Runx1-Runx1t1 after bone marrow transplantation. Ann Clin Pathol. 2014;2(1):1009.
33. Gamis AS, Alonzo TA, Meshinchi S, Sung L, Gerbing RB, Raimondi SC, et al. Gemtuzumab ozogamicin in children and adolescents with de novo acute myeloid leukemia improves event-free survival by reducing relapse risk: results from the randomized phase III Children's oncology group trial AAML0531. J Clin Oncol. 2014;32(27):3021–32.
34. Sievers EL, Larson RA, Stadtmauer EA, Estey E, Lowenberg B, Dombret H, et al. Efficacy and safety of gemtuzumab ozogamicin in patients with CD33-positive acute myeloid leukemia in first relapse. J Clin Oncol. 2001;19(13):3244–54.
35. Loken MR, Alonzo TA, Pardo L, Gerbing RB, Aplenc R, Sung L, et al. Multidimensional flow cytometry significantly improves upon the morphologic assessment of post-induction marrow remission status – comparison of morphology and multidimensional flow cytometry; a report from the Children's Oncology Group AML protocol AAML0531. Blood. 2011;118(21):939.
36. Loken MR, Alonzo TA, Pardo L, Gerbing RB, Aplenc R, Sung L, et al. Presence of residual disease detected by multidimensional flow cytometry identifies patients with AML at high risk

of relapse – a report from the Children's oncology group. Blood. 2011;118(21):3545.
37. Pongers-Willemse MJ, Verhagen OJ, Tibbe GJ, Wijkhuijs AJ, de Haas V, Roovers E, et al. Real-time quantitative PCR for the detection of minimal residual disease in acute lymphoblastic leukemia using junctional region specific TaqMan probes. Leukemia. 1998;12(12):2006–14.
38. ClinicalTrials.gov Bethesda, MD: National Institute of health; 2018 [cited 2018]. Available from: clinicaltrials.gov.

Chapter 5
ML-DS: A Unique Condition for Measurable Residual Disease Detection

Elisabeth R. Wilson and R. Spencer Tong

Introduction

The predisposition of children with Down syndrome (DS) toward developing acute leukemia has been well established. Interestingly, despite an approximate 500-fold increased risk of developing myeloid leukemia (ML) compared to their non-DS counterparts, children with ML-DS tend to respond favorably to treatment and experience increased survival rates [1]. Aside from demonstrating a consistent and overlapping megakaryocytic morphology with a subset of non-DS AML patients (FAB M7/AMKL), ML-DS patients lack any of the common cytogenetic aberrations or molecular diagnostic

---

E. R. Wilson (✉)
Hematologics Inc., Seattle, WA, USA

Washington University in St. Louis, Department of Biological and Biomedical Sciences, St. Louis, MO, USA
e-mail: wilsoner@wustl.edu

R. S. Tong
Washington University School of Medicine,
Department of Pediatrics, St. Louis, ON, USA

© Springer International Publishing AG,
part of Springer Nature 2019
T. E. Druley (ed.), *Minimal Residual Disease Testing*,
https://doi.org/10.1007/978-3-319-94827-0_5

markers used to diagnose and classify AML in non-DS individuals including AML-ETO, PML-RARA, t(15;17), MLL t(9;11), inv(16), etc. [2]. Rather, the most frequently observed cytogenetic abnormalities include trisomy 8, trisomy 11, del(6q), del(7p), del(16q), and dup(1p), wherein trisomy 8 has been the most significant cytogenetic abnormality associated with poor outcomes; however, the prognostic associations of trisomy 8 are still under investigation [3, 4]. Notably, those non-DS individuals with overlapping megakaryoblastic morphology consistently have the poorest treatment response and survival rates [5, 6], which is in clear contrast with favorable survival of DS-AML patients [7, 8]. The favorable survival characteristics of ML-DS, along with the advancing knowledge of its unique natural pathology, have necessitated a distinct disease classification from non-DS associated AML. As such, the well-founded prognostic system and outcome prediction models established for non-DS associated AML are not amenable to the treatment and monitoring of ML-DS.

To date, there is strong consensus regarding the natural history of ML-DS. Development of myeloid leukemia typically occurs before the age of 4 years and is typically preceded by preleukemic clonal expansion of the myeloid compartment during the neonatal period termed transient myeloproliferative disease (TMD) or transient abnormal myelopoiesis (TAM) [9, 10]. Among other clinical symptoms, TMD is characterized by the presence of circulating megakaryoblast cells encoding somatic N-terminal truncating mutations in the hematopoietic transcription factor *GATA1* [11, 12]. Acquisition of a truncating mutation resulting in the *GATA1* short form (GATA1s) product is predicted to occur in nearly all cases of TMD and is thought to be necessary, although not necessarily sufficient, for AML transformation [6, 13]. Because the majority of cases spontaneously resolve with a permanent remission within the first few months of birth, early intervention with low-intensity cytotoxic treatment is only considered where there is evidence of end-organ dysfunction. However, 20–30% of those patients with clinical TMD will go on to develop ML-DS before the age of 4, owing to the acquisition of addition somatic mutations in the GATA1s mutant containing clone [10, 14]. Patient response to therapy is collectively favorable with approximately 80% of patients achieving long-term remission after lower-intensity chemotherapy [1, 15, 16]. However, in the smaller subset of patients who fail to respond to upfront treatment, the propensity for relapse is high and is largely accompanied by an inability to achieve complete remission following relapse [16]. There remains little observed survival benefit for bone marrow transplant in the setting of relapse for children with ML-DS, and decision to pursue allogenic stem cell transplant is made with the knowledge of historically high failure rates [17]. While the general model of disease progression is well defined, the ability to predict which patients with TMD progress to ML-DS, and further which patients will eventually relapse, is still lacking.

Accordingly, a few significant challenges persist for physicians and scientists treating children with TMD and ML-DS. First, there remains a strong need to define a prognostic system that accurately predicts which patients are at risk of transforming from TMD to ML-DS, thereby enabling physicians to minimize treatment-related toxicity while leveraging risk-adapted treatment appropriately. Additionally, the field stands to gain a more extensive understanding of the germline and somatic mutation landscapes that drive transformation to ML-DS. Given that ML-DS clearly has a distinct etiology from non-DS childhood leukemia, a better understanding of the functional pathology may help inform a widely used prognostic system and will be increasingly relevant in devising individualized treatment approaches, both at diagnosis and for those patients who relapse.

Minimal residual disease (MRD) monitoring is the primary strategy used in the surveillance of pediatric leukemias to evaluate therapeutic efficacy and predict patient outcome. For over a decade, flow cytometric monitoring for residual disease has been the gold standard for detecting leukemia cells remaining in the marrow or peripheral blood following induction therapy, achieving levels of sensitivity and specificity to robustly identify leukemic cells at 1 in 1000 (0.1%) [18]. While currently the gold standard for residual disease detection, flow cytometry, is fundamentally limited by sample quality and by the propensity for antigenic shift, up to 90% of both adult and childhood AMLs will undergo immunophenotypic shift over the course of disease [19, 20]. In an era of high-throughput sequencing, the use of next-generation sequencing provides an attractive option for further increasing the sensitivity of detection, without the dependence on constant antigenic expression. Each approach presents with its own unique challenges, but the prospect of merging technologies for a more nuanced and comprehensive understanding of hematologic disease in the context of ML-DS presentation has gained traction among physicians and scientists.

Minimizing Treatment-Related Toxicity: Early Treatment Advances

In line with the challenge to minimize treatment-related toxicity, a number of clinical trials have been progressively designed to assess the possibility of reducing chemotherapy doses for ML-DS patients while maintaining favorable outcome rates. A Children's Cancer Group (CCG) trial, CCG 2891, conducted in the early 2000s highlighted the need to design specific treatment regimens for ML-DS patients. Administration of intensively timed treatment cycles of combined dexamethasone, cytarabine, 6-thioguanine, etoposide, and rubidomycin/daunomycin (DCTER) had previously been associated with improved survival rates in non-DS patients; however, applying the same treatment schedule to ML-DS patients leads to very high cytotoxic death rates (32%) [21]. In contrast, those ML-DS patients that received standard timing of DCTER cycles had lower rates of cytotoxic death (11%) which were more comparable to non-DS patients receiving the high-intensity treatment regimen [14].

Subsequently, the Children's Oncology Group (COG) conducted the first clinical trial designed to provide uniform treatment for myeloid leukemia tailored to ML-DS. Specifically, COG A2971 was a phase 3 clinical trial which sought to reduce the comorbidities and mortality rate in ML-DS patients by reducing treatment dose and eliminating maintenance therapy from the standard-timing regimen used in the previous CCG 2891 study. Elimination of etoposide and dexamethasone from the induction regimen and replacement of 3 months of maintenance chemotherapy with three intrathecal maintenance doses of cytarabine was sufficient, if not more effective, for maintaining increased overall survival rates (84% ± 6% in COG A2971 vs 79% ± 7% in CCG 2891) [22].

A recent 2017 report from an international ML-DS trial conducted by the Nordic Society for Pediatric Hematology and Oncology (NOPHO), Dutch Childhood Oncology Group (DCOG), and Acute Myeloid Leukemia-Berlin- Frankfurt-Münster (AML-BFM), demonstrated in the largest cohort to date that reduced treatment toxicity can still be accompanied by favorable survival rates. One hundred seventy ML-DS children were treated with reduced etoposide dosage, intrathecal central nervous system prophylaxis with cytarabine, and forewent maintenance therapy; the 5-year survival for these children did not differ significantly from the historical control arm [4]. It is also important to note that while the group was able to demonstrate that reducing therapy does not hinder exceptional outcomes in these children, the identification of clear prognostic factors predicting which patients were at risk for relapse and in need of intensive therapy remained indefinable.

Multidimensional Flow Cytometry in ML-DS Treatment and Residual Disease Monitoring

Until recently, the use of morphologic bone marrow assessment has been the main determinant of clinical response to treatment for AML patients—serving as a primary measurement to advise further patient treatment. In the past two decades, multidimensional flow cytometry (MDF) has replaced morphologic assessment as the gold standard for residual disease monitoring in hematologic malignancy due to its heightened sensitivity and specificity in detecting rare clonal populations of cells that may be consistent with persistent disease. In multiple prospective, multicenter clinical trials, MDF detection of MRD has proven to be an independent predictor of outcome in lymphoblastic and myeloid leukemias [19, 23–29]. The MDF strategy employed in a number of COG clinical trials is termed "difference from normal (ΔN)" and is predicated on a detailed understanding of global cell surface antigen expression during each stage of hematologic development from an HSC to a given lineage-specific cell type. Thus, ΔN MDF detects cell populations that deviate from normal developmental surface immunophenotypes and has been shown to more accurately predict patient outcomes where morphological assessment either fails to detect residual disease or inaccurately classifies patients with heightened, but normal, blast counts as having persistent disease. Quantification and correlation of cell surface antigens expression allow for an assessment of general specimen composition, as well as robust identification of populations with aberrant expression phenotypes that may be consistent with residual disease. Further, ΔN analysis diverges from the commonly used leukemia-associated immunophenotyping (LAIP) owing to its lack of dependence on a diagnostic reference. For more specifics on the ΔN approach, please see Chap. 4.

While the ΔN MDF approach has been validated in multiple prospective COG AML trials, the use of MDF in the setting of ML-DS has not reached the same level of significance until the most recent clinical trials, largely because quantitative characterization of normal and abnormal surface immunophenotypes during developmental hematopoiesis in DS individuals has been lacking.

A 2017 report from the COG was issued with results from the AAML0431 clinical trial, which was designed to build upon and improve the favorable outcome results that were observed with reduced chemotherapy doses. AAML0431 consisted of four cycles of induction and two cycles of intensification therapy based on the treatment schema of the previous COG A2971 trial with several modifications. In brief, high-dose cytarabine (HD-araC) was administered in a second induction cycle instead of the intensification cycle, and one of four daunorubicin-containing induction cycles was eliminated. Of particular significance, AAML0431 was the first trial to identify MRD as prognostic factor for ML-DS patients [30]. Amidst a number of factors assessed for prognostic significance in correlative biological studies, flow cytometric assessment of MRD at day 28 post-induction I was the only significant predictor of outcome in both univariable and multivariable analyses. The 5-year DFS for MRD-negative patients was 92.7% vs 76.2% for MRD-positive patients [19].

On the newly established basis that MRD status by flow cytometry provides a robust prognostic variable, an ongoing international phase 3 prospective study for ML-DS was launched by COG in 2016 entitled: "Risk-stratified Therapy for Acute Myeloid Leukemia in Down Syndrome" (AAML1531). This study will aim to enroll 240 ML-DS patients with a therapeutic aim of determining whether outstanding event-free and overall survival could be achieved without the use of high-dose cytarabine (HD Ara-C) for standard-risk patients as indicated by post-induction MRD status. Briefly, treatment groups are determined based on flow cytometric MRD status following induction therapy wherein standard-risk patients are classified under the criteria of having low MRD (less than 0.05%), while high-risk patients are classified under the criteria of having increased MRD (greater than or equal to 0.05%). As outcome data from the AAML1531 trial matures, the efficacy of the risk-adapted treatment based on flow cytometric MDR assessment will become clearer.

To date, these studies as well as number case reports have revealed the consistency of leukemic antigen expression associated with ML-DS marked by expression of CD33 (+)/CD13 (+/−)/CD38 (+)/CD117 (+)/CD34 (+/−)/CD7 (+)/CD56

(+/−)/CD36 (+)/CD71 (+)/CD42b (+)/HLA-DR (+/−) [31]. Not only does there appear to be reduced heterogeneity in diagnostic immunophenotypes for this cohort, the ML-DS immunophenotype is unique from common immunophenotypes observed in DS patients with later onset of AML (after the age of 4) (Fig. 5.1), which are considered to be a separate disease entity more consistent with non-DS AMKL cases [32]. Few studies have addressed the landscape of antigen expression observed during post-chemotherapy follow-up in the DS patient cohort, and perhaps highlighting a greater deficiency, even fewer studies have characterized and quantified the immunophenotypic patterns of normal hematopoietic development in DS individuals.

In one recent study that assessed follow-up ML-DS specimens for residual disease using the ΔN approach, 98% of specimens ($n = 144/147$) from 48 individuals had suspicious

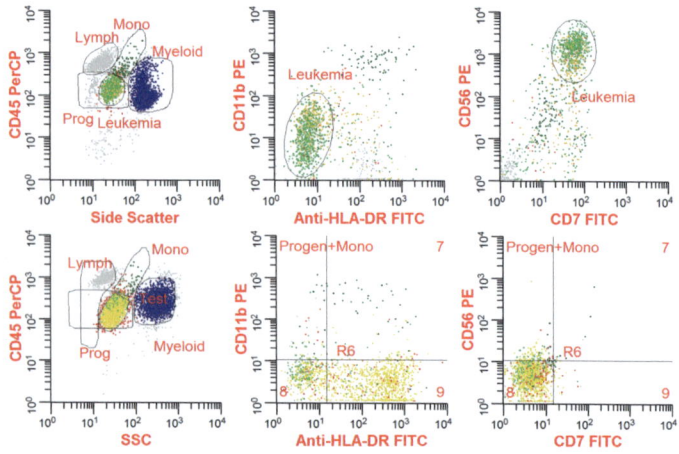

FIGURE 5.1 Representative DS-AML diagnostic immunophenotype. Top: example of distinguishing parameters in the recurring diagnostic phenotype for DS-AML (<4 years old). Bottom: similar parameters of common diagnostic phenotype for AML in DS individuals >4 years old. The leukemia is shown in bright green (top) or gold (bottom). CD34 positive cells are is shown in bright green and gold, lymphocytes are shown in gray, mono-cytes in dark green, and myeloid cells in blue. Adapted from Wilson ER. [33]

CD34+ progenitor populations that expressed CD56 and/or lacked HLA-DR at one or more follow-up time points (Fig. 5.2) [33]. Of note, these CD34+/CD56+/HLA-DR-cells were only partially overlapping with the diagnostic immunophenotype. In each case reported to be MRD negative, the CD34+/CD56+/HLA-DR-cells lacked the CD7 expression observed on the diagnostic clone. Interestingly, in three DS patients undergoing treatment for B-cell acute lymphoblastic leukemia (B-ALL), the same immunophenotypic features (CD34+/CD56+/HLA-DR) were observed in myeloblasts

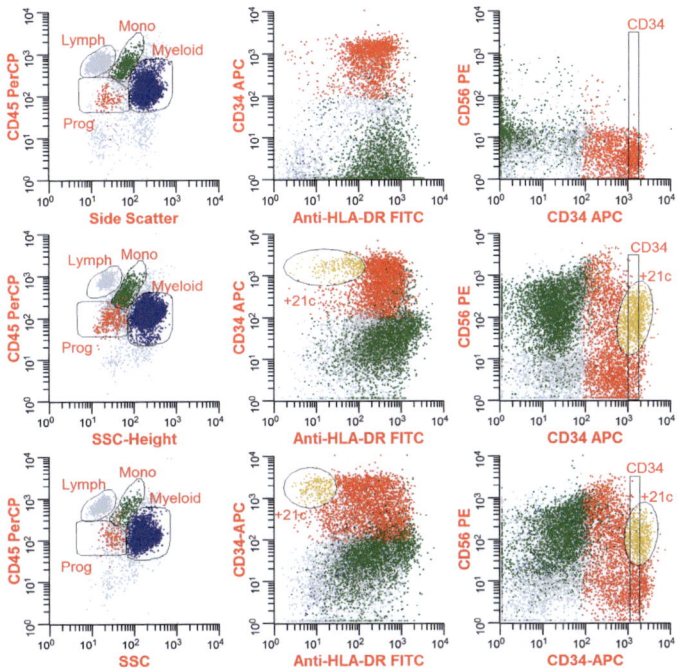

FIGURE 5.2 Comparison of post-induction chemotherapy regeneration in BM for non-DS AML (top panel), DS-AML (middle panel), and DS-ALL (bottom panel). CD34 progenitors are colored in red, while the DS-associated myeloid progenitors, which co-express CD56 and CD34, are colored in gold. Lymphocytes are shown in gray, monocytes in dark green, and myeloid cells in blue. Adapted from Wilson ER. [33]

from bone marrow specimens harvested after chemotherapy (Fig. 5.2) [34]. The remarkable consistency of this post-chemotherapy immunophenotype across the two diseases, along with the well-documented increased survival rates of ML-DS patients, questions whether these CD34+/CD56+/HLA-DR- progenitors are truly persistent leukemic cells or perhaps are representative of a nonmalignant regenerative population inherent to hematopoiesis in a trisomic 21 background.

In the same study, progenitor cell populations in post-chemotherapy specimens were sorted and further assessed for the presence of diagnostic molecular markers in a subset of patients. In brief, fluorescence-activated cell sorting (FACS) of the CD34+ cells with CD56 expression was performed on five individual specimens for subsequent FISH or SNP/CGH microarray to assess for overlap with the diagnostic ML-DS clone. In all five cases, features of the diagnostic leukemic clone were not observed in the sorted cells (Table 5.1), further supporting the hypothesis that these CD56+ progenitor populations may be more consistent with normal regenerating myeloid populations rather than persistent disease.

It has been reported that granulocytes and monocytes from DS patients frequently express CD56 in stressed bone marrow such as post-chemotherapy or inflammation [34, 35]. This preliminary study extends the observation to regenerating myeloblasts in DS patients. CD56 is not expressed on normal myeloblasts and is a marker frequently used for assessing blast aberrancy in MDF. As the leukemic myeloblasts in Down syndrome frequently express CD56 and CD7 with concomitant loss of HLA-DR, it is important to recognize the unusual expression pattern of regenerating myeloblasts, particularly for those utilizing the LAIP approach. As the current difference from normal approach is based on an understanding of myeloblast immunophenotype in individuals with normal karyotypes, new algorithms need to be developed and validated with respect to the immunophenotype of normal myeloblasts from Down syndrome patients.

Chapter 5. DS-AML: A Unique Condition for MRD 149

TABLE 5.1 Genotypic analysis of the DS-associated myeloid progenitor cells in regenerating, post-chemotherapy bone marrow. In five DS-AML patient cases, cell sorting (FACS) of the DS-associated myeloid progenitor population was completed. In all five cases, the diagnostic genetic clone was not observed in the sorted cells

Patient #	Frequency of DS associated myeloid population (34+/56+)	Sorted cell fraction	Leukemic diagnostic genotype	Genetic assessment of sorted fraction
1	0.4% total non-erythroid cells	CD34+	Trisomy 8	No evidence of trisomy 8 by FISH (D8Z2 probe) in 34 analyzed interphases
2	0.4% total non-erythroid cells	CD34+	Trisomy 8	No evidence of trisomy 8 by FISH (D8Z2 probe) in 200 analyzed interphases
3	0.08% total non-erythroid cells	CD34+/CD56+	Trisomy 8	No evidence of trisomy 8 by FISH (AML1/ETO probe) in 66 analyzed interphases
4	0.04% total non-erythroid cells	CD34+/CD56+	Gain of 11q	No evidence of gain of 11q by FISH in 27 analyzed interphases
5	0.1% total non-erythroid cells	CD34+/CD56+	5q deletion	No evidence of 5q deletion by aCGH/SNP microarray

Making Sense of the Somatic Mutation Landscapes: Leveraging Error-Corrected NGS

While ΔN MDF for MRD monitoring has improved risk stratification in ML-DS, its theoretical efficacy is limited by the reproducibility and interpretation of the data between institutions and by the high frequency with which individual patient's leukemias undergo antigenic shift. While more robust MRD detection platforms are needed, this demand is exacerbated in ML-DS as MRD measurements by ΔN MDF were negative in approximately half of all ML-DS patients who relapsed on the AAML0431 study by the COG [36].

MRD assessment by next-generation sequencing (NGS) offers a versatile detection platform that may supplement— or eventually supplant—conventional ΔN MDF screening. With its ability to survey billions of DNA nucleotides in a single sequencing run, NGS can identify molecular signatures and track mutational shifts between diagnosis and relapse. However, NGS faces its own technical limit of detection due to errors introduced during library preparation and sequencing. With a documented error rate of 1–1.5%, the detection of rare somatic mutations below a 2% variant allele fraction (VAF) requires costly and time-intensive resequencing [37–39]. Several groups have developed error-corrected sequencing (ECS) methods to address these limitations and circumvent the NGS error rate [40]. Error-corrected sequencing involves tagging individual DNA molecules with unique oligonucleotide indexes through ligation or hybridization approaches. Following PCR amplification, sequence reads with the same index are grouped into read families. Consensus sequences are built by comparing reads within said read families and subsequently removing sequencing errors unshared between reads. Consensus sequences are then aligned to each other and a reference genome for mutation calling [41, 42]. These technological advances have lowered the limit of detection of NGS by two orders of magnitude; ECS can confidently call and characterize mutations at a level of 1 mutant cell per 10,000 wild-type cells. Error-corrected NGS is therefore a viable alternative MRD platform with its identical limit of detection to ΔN MDF, is not limited by epitope evolution, and can identify and track mutations throughout disease progression.

Given the previous lack of known, consistent cell surface markers for leukemic blasts in DS patients, the variability in genetic lesions, and the limited diagnostic samples obtained in many cases due to preceding myelodysplasia, there currently exists no bona fide method of MRD detection for ML-DS. However, it has been well-documented that this unique leukemia and its preleukemic condition, TMD, are rooted in the acquisition of somatic mutations in the *GATA1* transcription factor [43]. This X-linked gene is crucial in hematopoietic development and exhibits distinct regulation on erythropoiesis and megakaryopoiesis. Early mouse models from Stuart Orkin's group demonstrated that *GATA1*-null animals died from anemia during embryogenesis and that erythroid progenitors apoptose prematurely [44, 45]. Interestingly, the opposite effect is seen as loss of *GATA1* prevents terminal differentiation of megakaryocytes [46]. These findings led to the work of John Crispino's group which provided evidence that mutations in *GATA1* are defining events in the pathogenesis of ML-DS [47]. Since then, numerous studies have been published profiling the incidence of mutations in exons 2 and 3 of *GATA1* in children with both ML-DS and TMD at >85% of cases [48, 49]. Though the molecular mechanisms of leukemic transformation in ML-DS remain to be elucidated, there's no doubt that acquired mutations in *GATA1* are an essential step in the pathogenesis of this unique leukemia. Quite like ΔN MDF for the distinct immunophenotypes of ML-DS, *GATA1* mutations appear to be a suitable biomarker for targeted ECS for MRD detection in ML-DS.

While the cooperation of trisomy 21 and a truncated GATA1s protein are necessary for leukemogenesis, these two events are not sufficient for disease [50]. This is demonstrated by a report by Irene Roberts and colleagues showing that 30% of DS neonates, without overt hematologic abnormalities, are born with a detectable *GATA1* mutation [51]. While this study exemplifies the striking, yet inexplicable, link between trisomy 21 and *GATA1*, it also shows that ML-DS transformation requires other cooperating mutations. Lending further support to this disease model is a study by Kenichi Yoshida and colleagues who published a robust genomic characterization of ML-DS and TMD patients. They provided additional evidence that while TMD may be caused by constitutive trisomy 21 and a *GATA1* mutation alone, progression to ML-DS requires the acquisition of recurrent somatic mutations in the cohesion complex, *CTCF,* epigenetic regulators, and more [52] These findings are important in understanding the biology of ML-DS, as well as for the development of technologies that can appropriately detect residual disease. Despite lacking the evidence to support this disease model in vivo, one can envision that an error-corrected sequencing panel targeting *GATA1* and these recurrently cooperating mutations would be immensely valuable in not only understanding TMD evolution but for MRD detection as well.

Conclusions and Future Outlook

MRD detection in ML-DS has significantly improved with the advent of multidimensional flow cytometry; however, our incomplete knowledge of the normal immunophenotype of hematopoietic DS cells has limited the theoretical efficiency of the established ΔN MDF method. While clinical trial groups like the Children's Oncology Group continue to refine risk stratification based on these technologies, next-generation sequencing has emerged as a novel candidate platform for MRD detection.

ML-DS is almost ubiquitously characterized by mutations in the *GATA1* transcription factor. While the full etiology of ML-DS from its preleukemic condition TMD is not fully understood, targeted NGS for *GATA1* mutations as an MRD method is an appropriate base. With its ability to identify and track mutations between leukemic presentation and relapse, NGS offers a solution for the mutational and antigenic instability plaguing this disease. Moreover, NGS will allow for the broad characterization of the clonal heterogeneity in healthy DS children which will distinguish benign clonal hematopoiesis from a pre-ML-DS state. This will lead to the construction of more exhaustive NGS panels targeting recurrent mutations in ML-DS transformation and relapse beyond *GATA1*.

Error-corrected sequencing addresses the sensitivity limitations of conventional NGS through unique molecular indices and bioinformatic correction. ECS leverages the flexibility and characterization potential of NGS with the putative sensitivity of ΔN MDF. Though future studies will be required to confirm its utility for MRD detection in ML-DS, the union of ECS with the speed and throughput of ΔN MDF promises for a deeper understanding of this distinctive leukemia and its mechanisms for relapse.

References

1. Creutzig U, Reinhardt D, Diekamp S, Dworzak M, Stary J, Zimmermann M. AML patients with down syndrome have a high cure rate with AML-BFM therapy with reduced dose intensity. Leukemia. 2005;19(8):1355–60.
2. Blink M, et al. Normal karyotype is a poor prognostic factor in myeloid leukemia of down syndrome: a retrospective, international study. Haematologica. 2014;99:299–307.
3. Forestier E, et al. Cytogenetic features of acute lymphoblastic and myeloid leukemias in pediatric patients with down syndrome: an iBFM-SG study. Blood. 2008;111:1575–83.
4. Uffmann M, et al. Therapy reduction in patients with down syndrome and myeloid leukemia: the international ML-DS 2006 trial. Blood. 2017;129(25):3314–21.
5. Hama A, Yagasaki H, Takahashi Y, et al. Acute megakaryoblastic leukaemia (AMKL) in children: a comparison of AMKL with and without down syndrome. Br J Haematol. 2008;140:552–61.

6. Barnard DR, Alonzo TA, Gerbing RB, Lange B, Woods WG. Comparison of childhood myelodysplastic syndrome, AML FAB M6 or M7, CCG 2891: report from the Children's Oncology Group. Pediatr Blood Cancer. 2007;49:17–22.
7. Athale UH, et al. Biology and outcome of childhood acute megakaryoblastic leukemia: a single institution's experience. Blood. 2001;97(12):3727–32.
8. Inaba H, et al. Heterogeneous cytogenetic subgroups and outcomes in childhood acute megakaryoblastic leukemia: a retrospective international study. Blood. 2015;126:1575–84.
9. Roberts I, Izraeli S. Haematopoietic development and leukaemia in down syndrome. Br J Haematol. 2014;167(5):587–99.
10. Bhatnagar N, et al. Transient abnormal Myelopoiesis and AML in down syndrome: an update. Curr Hematol Malig Rep. 2016;11:333–41.
11. Maligne S, Izraeli S, Crispino JD. Insights into the manifestations, outcomes and mechanisms of leukemogenesis in down syndrome. Blood. 2009;113(12):2610–28.
12. Hitzler JK, Cheung J, Li Y, Scherer SW, Zipursky A. *GATA1* mutations in transient leukemia and acute megakaryoblastic leukemia of down syndrome. Blood. 2003;101:4301–4.
13. Gamis AS, Alonzo T, Gerbing R, Hildren J, et al. Natural history of transient myeloproliferative disorder clinically diagnosed in down syndrome neonates: a report from the Children's Oncology Group Study A2971. Blood. 2011;118:6752–9.
14. Greene ME, et al. Mutations in *GATA1* in both transient myeloproliferative disorder and acute megakaryoblastic leukemia of down syndrome. Blood Cell Mol Dis. 2003;31(3):351–6.
15. Kudo K, Kojima S, Tabuchi K, Yabe H, Tawa A, Imaizumi M, et al. Prospective study of a Pirarubicin, intermediate-dose Cytarabine, and etoposide regimen in children with down syndrome and acute myeloid leukemia: the Japanese childhood AML Cooperative Study Group. J Clin Oncol. 2007;25(34):5442–7.
16. Taga T, et al. Clinical characteristics and outcome of refractory/relapsed myeloid leukemia in children with down syndrome. Blood. 2012;120(9):1810–5.
17. Hitzler JK, et al. Outcome of transplantation for acute myelogenous leukemia in children with down syndrome. Biol Blood Marrow Transplant. 2013;19(6):893–7.
18. Loken, et al. Residual disease detected by multidimensional flow cytometry signifies high relapse risk in patients with de novo acute myeloid leukemia: a report from Children's Oncology Group. Blood. 2012;120(8):1581–8.

19. Sievers EL, et al. Immunophenotypic evidence of leukemia after induction therapy predicts relapse: results from a prospective Children's Cancer Group Study of 252 patients with acute myeloid leukemia. Blood. 2003;101(9):3398–406.
20. Baer MR, et al. High frequency of immunophenotype changes in acute myeloid leukemia at relapse: implications for residual disease detection (Cancer and Leukemia Group B Study 8361). Blood. 2001;97(11):3574–80.
21. Gamis AS, et al. Increased age at diagnosis has a significantly negative effect on outcome in children with down syndrome and acute myeloid leukemia: a report from the Children's Cancer Group Study 2891. J Clin Oncol. 2003;21:3415–22.
22. Sorrell AD, et al. Favorable survival maintained in children who have myeloid leukemia associated with down syndrome using reduced-dose chemotherapy on Children's Oncology Group trial A2971: a report from the Children's Oncology Group. Cancer. 2012;118(19):4806.
23. Rubnitz JE, et al. Minimal residual disease-directed therapy for childhood acute myeloid leukaemia: results of the AML02 multicentre trial. Lancet Oncol. 2010;11(6):543–52.
24. Cooper TM, et al. AAML03P1, a pilot study of the safety of gemtuzumab ozogamicin in combination with chemotherapy for newly diagnosed childhood acute myeloid leukemia: a report from the Children's Oncology Group. Cancer. 2012;118(3):76–769.
25. Loken MR, et al. Multidimensional flow cytometry significantly improves upon the morphologic assessment of post-induction marrow remission status—comparison of morphology and multidimensional flow cytometry: a report from the Children's Oncology Group AML protocol AAML0531 [abstract]. Blood (ASH Annual Meeting Abstracts). 2011;118(21). Abstract):939.
26. Basso G, et al. Risk of relapse of childhood acute lymphoblastic leukemia is predicted by flow cytometric measurement of residual disease on day 15 bone marrow. J Clin Oncol. 2009;27(31):5168–74.
27. Denys B, et al. Improved flow cytometric detection of minimal residual disease in childhood acute lymphoblastic leukemia. Leukemia. 2013;27(3):635–41.
28. Borowitz MJ, et al. Clinical significance of minimal residual disease in childhood acute lymphoblastic leukemia and its relationship to other prognostic factors: a Children's Oncology Group study. Blood. 2008;111:5477–85.

29. Walter R, et al. Significance of minimal residual disease before myeloablative allogeneic hematopoietic cell transplantation for AML in first and second complete remission. Blood. 2013;122(18):1813.
30. Taub JW, et al. Improved outcomes for myeloid leukemia of don syndrome: a report from the Children's Oncology Group AAML0431 trial. Blood. 2017;129(25):3304–13.
31. Langebrake C, et al. Immunophenotype of down syndrome acute myeloid leukemia and transient myeloproliferative disease differs significantly from other diseases with morphologically identical or similar blasts. Klin Padiatr. 2005;217:126–34.
32. Bourquin JP, et al. Identification of distinct molecular phenotypes in acute megakaryoblastic leukemia by gene expression profiling. Proc Natl Acad Sci USA. 2006;103:3339–44.
33. Wilson ER, et al. Down syndrome AML is unique in phenotype both at diagnosis and in post chemotherapy regeneration. Blood (ASH Annual Meeting Abstracts). 2016;128(22):1687.
34. Langebrake C, Klusmann JH, Wortmann K, Kolar M, Puhlmann U, Reinhardt D. Concomitant aberrant overexpression of RUNX1 and NCAM in regenerating bone marrow of myeloid leukemia of Down's syndrome. Haematologica. 2006;91(11):1473–80.
35. Karandikar NJ, Aquino DB, McKenna RW, Kroft SH. Transient myeloproliferative disorder and acute myeloid leukemia in down syndrome - an immunophenotypic analysis. Am J Clin Pathol. 2001;116(2):204–10.
36. Taub J, et al. Minimal residual disease (MRD) identifies down syndrome acute myeloid leukemia (DS-AML) patients with extremely high event free survival (EFS) rates: results of the Children's Oncology Group (COG) phase III AAML0431 trial. Blood (ASH annual meeting abstracts). 2014;124:278.
37. Manley LJ, et al. Monitoring error rates in Illumina sequencing. J Biomol Tech. 2016;4:125–8.
38. Shendure J, Ji H. Next-generation DNA sequencing. Nat Biotechnol. 2008;26:1135–45.
39. Quail MA, et al. A large genome center's improvements to the Illumina sequencing system. Nat Methods. 2008;5:1005–10.
40. Young AL, et al. Quantifying ultra-rare pre-leukemic clones via targeted error-corrected sequencing. Leukemia. 2015;29:1608–11.
41. Wong TN, et al. Role of TP53 mutations in the origin and evolution of therapy-related acute myeloid leukaemia. Nature. 2015;518:552–5.

42. Young AL, et al. Clonal hematopoiesis harbouring AML-associated mutations is ubiquitous in healthy adults. Nat Commun. 2016;7:12484.
43. Crispino JD. *GATA1* in normal and malignant hematopoiesis. Semin Cell Dev Biol. 2005;16:137–47.
44. Martin DI, Orkin SH. Transcriptional activation and DNA binding by the erythroid factor GF-1/NF-E1/Eryf 1. Genes Dev. 1990;4(11):1886–98.
45. Fujiwara Y, et al. Arrested development of embryonic red cell precursors in mouse embryos lacking transcription factor GATA-1. Proc Natl Acad Sci USA. 1996;93(22):12355–8.
46. Crispino JD, Horwitz MS. GATA factor mutations in hematologic disease. Blood. 2017;129(15):2103–10.
47. Wechsler J, et al. Acquired mutations in *GATA1* in the megakaryoblastic leukemia of down syndrome. Nat Genet. 2002;32:148–52.
48. Alford KA, et al. Analysis of *GATA1* mutations in down syndrome transient myeloproliferative disorder and myeloid leukemia. Blood. 2011;118(8):2222–38.
49. Kanezaki R, et al. Down syndrome and *GATA1* mutations in transient abnormal myeloproliferative disorder: mutation classes correlate with progression to myeloid leukemia. Blood. 2010;116(22):4631–8.
50. Malinge S, et al. Increased dosage of the chromosome 21 ortholog *Dyrk1a* promotes megakaryoblastic leukemia in a murine model of down syndrome. J Clin Invest. 2012;122(3):948–62.
51. Roberts I, et al. *GATA1*-mutant clones are frequent and often unsuspected in babies with down syndrome: identification of a population at risk of leukemia. Blood. 2013;122(24):3908–17.
52. Yoshida K, et al. The landscape of somatic mutations in down syndrome-related myeloid disorders. Nat Genet. 2013;45:1293–9.

Chapter 6
Advancements in Next-Generation Sequencing for Detecting Minimal Residual Disease

Erin L. Crowgey and Nitin Mahajan

Introduction

The sequencing of DNA molecules enables the precise identification and order of nucleotides. These techniques include any method or technology that is used to determine the order of the four bases—adenine (A), guanine (G), cytosine (C), and thymine (T)—in a strand of DNA. Massively parallel sequencing, also known as next-generation sequencing (NGS),

DNA is a giant resource that will change mankind, like the printing press.
– James D. Watson [1]

E. L. Crowgey (✉)
Nemours Alfred I. duPont Hospital for Children, Biomedical Research Department, Wilmington, DE, USA
e-mail: erin.crowgey@nemours.org

N. Mahajan
Washington University in St. Louis, Pediatric Hematology and Oncology, St Louis, MO, USA

© Springer International Publishing AG,
part of Springer Nature 2019
T. E. Druley (ed.), *Minimal Residual Disease Testing*,
https://doi.org/10.1007/978-3-319-94827-0_6

is a method of simultaneously sequencing millions of fragments of DNA (or complementary DNA) simultaneously. These advancements have revolutionized the field of molecular biology [2–4] and are routinely used in a wide variety of research and clinical settings. Indispensable knowledge attained with modern DNA sequencing technology has been instrumental to unveil the plethora of previously hidden facts not only in the medical field but also in plant biology, forensic science, and evolution [3, 5].

Since the inexplicable relationship between genetic instability and tumorigenesis was proposed by Nowell in 1976 [6], progress in cancer genomics has strengthened and provided strong evidence to support this fundamental hypothesis. Most genetic disorders have been associated with modifications within regions that affect the coding of proteins, and are often divided into three types of categories: (1) single-gene disorder, (2) chromosomal disorders, and (3) complex disorders. There are many challenges associated with characterizing a genetic disorder, creating a unique niche for developing appropriate bioinformatics methodologies.

New developments in molecular biology techniques, which are often used to gain insight into genetic disorders, are generating massive amounts of data that need processed and refined prior to being incorporated into electronic health records (EHR) or clinical decision support applications [7]. Although these new techniques, such as NGS, are gaining momentum in the clinical field, there are no gold standards for clinical data analysis, interpretation, and integration that can be broadly applied to all disorders. Technical advancements in NGS led to a dramatic decrease in sequencing costs, mostly due to increase in the volume of data generated over the same period of time, to the point where an entire human genome in 2018 can be sequenced for less than $1000 [8], which ultimately increases its accessibility to researchers. Unfortunately, this expansion in data production has not been accompanied by an equivalent improvement in sequencing fidelity, as the chemistry needed for speed and volume currently comes at the price of precision, which is of little consequence when looking for sequence changes that are heterozygous or homozygous. To be clear, no amount of "deep sequencing" will be able to recover true mutations occurring at frequencies below the error rate of the sequencing platform itself as stochastic errors are continually generated at a constant rate [9]. Yet, the promise of genome-driven information in medical science is undoubtedly inspiring as witnessed by the targeted therapies based on the detection of oncogenic drivers [10, 11].

The corollary to the volumes of sequence data generated is the necessity for subsequent computational strategies to handle the previously incomprehensible volumes of data. Ultimately, there is a unique niche in the informatics field, especially in bioinformatics, to develop and deliver robust methodologies capable of analyzing the massive amount of data being generated by new technologies. Bioinformatics, an interdisciplinary field, requires the intersection of computer science, statistics, mathematics, biology, and engineering, with the ultimate goal of being applied in the clinical field for translating large biological datasets into diagnostic or predictive knowledge, clearly requiring a team science approach.

In Table 6.1, we list a brief history of the advances and applications of DNA (cDNA) sequencing techniques, as well as bioinformatic analyses, along with their applicability and challenges in detecting the minimal residual disease (MRD) in leukemia patients, which is highlighted in Table 6.2.

Cancer Genetics

The French-American-British (FAB) classification is a morphology-based system that was introduced several decades ago to help classify specific leukemias into subgroups [12]. Unfortunately, throughout the last several years, it has become apparent that a general classification system, such as FAB, does not apply broadly and appropriately apply to all cancer types and age ranges, as the genetic landscape between adult and pediatric cancers can be much different [13].

TABLE 6.1 History Ssequencing

Year	Lead researcher/ association	Highlight
1865	Gregor Mendel	Uses peas to figure out the fundamental of principles of heredity
1871	Friedrich Miescher	Identified the presence of "nuclein" (now known as DNA) and associated proteins, in the cell nucleus
1904	Walter Sutton and Theodor Boveri	Proposed the chromosome theory of heredity after finding that chromosomes occur in matched pairs, one inherited from the mother and one from the father
1910	Albrecht Kossel	Discovered the five nucleotide bases, adenine, cytosine, guanine, thymine, and uracil
1950	Erwin Chargaff	Suggested pairing pattern of the bases A, C, G, and T
1952	Alfred Hershey and Martha Chase	Demonstrated DNA, rather than protein, carries genetic information
1953	James Watson and Francis Crick	Published the double helix structure of DNA
1961	Marshall Nirenberg, Har Gobind Khorana, and colleagues	Identified how to read the DNA sequences in blocks of three "codon." Each codon codes for an amino acid which is added to the protein during translation
1965	Robert Holley and colleagues	Sequenced yeast tRNA
1970	Ray Wu	Used primer extension to read a short sequence of DNA for the first time
1972	Walter Fiers	Sequenced first whole gene coding for a MS2 virus protein
1973	Walter Gilbert and Allan Maxam	Developed a method to sequence DNA using chemicals to cut DNA at certain bases

TABLE 6.1 (continued)

Year	Lead researcher/ association	Highlight
1975	Frederick Sanger	Introduced "plus and minus" method for DNA sequencing using gels to separate DNA by size
1977	Frederick Sanger	Establishes dideoxy sequencing methodology
1983	Kary Mullis	Developed polymerase chain reaction (PCR)
1984	Fritz Pohl	Developed nonradioactive sequencing platform
1985	Alec Jeffreys	Developed a method for DNA profiling
1986	Leray Hoad and Applied Biosystem (ABI)	Developed first automated sequencer
1990	Human Genome Project (world's largest collaborative biological project)	Human Genome Project is launched
1995	Fleischmann RD and colleagues	Bacterial genome sequenced (*Haemophilus influenzae*)
	Fraser CM and colleagues	Bacterial genome sequenced (*Mycoplasma genitalium*)
1996	Mostafa Ronaghi	Introduced pyrosequencing, next-generation "sequencing by synthesis" method
	Applied Biosystem (ABI)	Introduced first commercial sequencing using capillary electrophoresis
	International collaboration	Sequenced the genome of yeast, *Saccharomyces cerevisiae*

(continued)

TABLE 6.1 (continued)

Year	Lead researcher/ association	Highlight
1998	John Sulston and Bob Waterston	Published the genome of the nematode worm, *Caenorhabditis elegans*
	Solexa Inc.	Developed sequencing by synthesis method that uses fluorescent dye
1999	Part of Human Genome Project	First human chromosome 22 is sequenced
2000		Genome of *Drosophila melanogaster* sequenced
	University of California, Santa Cruz	Launch of the UCSC Genome Browser
2001	Human Genome Project	Human Genome Project publishes first draft human genome sequence
2002	International Mouse Genome Sequencing Consortium	Mouse genome published
	The International HapMap Project	Project is launched to generate a "catalogue" of common human genetic variations and their locations
2003	Human Genome Project	Completed and confirmed humans have approximately 20,000–25,000 genes
	National Human Genome Research Institute	Launched the ENCODE project with the aims to identify and characterize all the genes in the human genome
2005	454 Life Sciences	The 454 system, based on pyrosequencing becomes the first commercially available next-generation sequencer

TABLE 6.1 (continued)

Year	Lead researcher/ association	Highlight
	The International HapMap Project	Map of human genetic variations published
2007	SOLid Systems	Launched a sequencing technology based on ligation
2008	1000 Genomes Project	Aims to sequence the whole genomes of a large number of people (2500)
	Cancer Genome Consortium	Comprehensive analysis of cancer genome
	Ley TJ	Sequences first cancer (AML) genome characterized by NGS
2009		Third-generation sequencing with single-molecule fluorescence technology is launched with Helicos sequencer
2011	Pacific Biosciences	Launched first commercial single-molecule real-time technology
2012	Oxford Nanopore Technologies	Commercialization of the portable nanopore sequencing methods

In 1976, Nowell highlighted the strong relationship between genetic instability and tumorigenesis [6], which provided the foundation for studying precise genetic alterations and their association with cancer. The majority of genetic analyses for cancer have been conducted using traditional cytogenetic techniques, such as karyotyping, and cytogenetic markers have played a major role in the diagnosis and classification of leukemias. The field of cytogenetics was initiated in 1956 [14] with the discovery and description of the number of chromosomes in a diploid human cell. There are several different techniques within the cytogenetic field that have been previously reviewed [15]. Overall, sensitivity and specificity are optimized when multiple cytogenetic methods are performed concurrently to overcome the limitations of any single method. Therefore, it is essential to have broad and precise methods to integrate multiple data sources for characterizing MRD to facilitate risk stratification and therapeutic selection [16].

History of DNA Sequencing

In 1910, Albrecht Kossel discovered the five nucleotide bases: adenine, cytosine, guanine, thymine and uracil, as the fundamental building blocks of nucleic acids [17]. Four decades later, Erin Chargaff recognized the pairing pattern of these nucleotides in DNA and RNA [17]. Robert Holley and colleagues (1965) were accredited for sequencing the first ever full nucleic acid molecule, 77 nucleotides of the yeast, *Saccharomyces cerevisiae*, alanine tRNA with a proposed cloverleaf structure [18]. It took more than 5 years to extract enough tRNA from the yeast to identify the sequence of nucleotide residues using specific ribonucleases, two-dimensional chromatography, and spectrophotometric procedures [18]. Initially, scientists focused their sequencing efforts on the readily available populations of RNA species because of the following properties: (i) bulk production in culture, (ii) not complicated by a complementary strand, and (iii) considerably shorter than DNA [19, 20]. The laborious and expensive nature of the sequencing drove the continuous development and refinement of subsequent sequencing methods.

Fred Sanger and colleagues at Cambridge were also actively working on methods for sequencing DNA molecules. They developed a technique based on the detection of radio-labeled partially-digested fragments after two-dimensional fractionation [21], allowing addition of nucleotides to the growing pool of ribosomal and transfer RNA sequences. Using a primer extension method in year 1968, Ray Wu and Dale Kaiser sequenced a short sequence of DNA for the first time [22]. However, the actual determination of bases was still restricted to small sequences of DNA because of the requirement for radioactive and hazardous chemicals. These continuous efforts resulted in generating the first complete protein-coding gene sequence, which was the coat protein of bacteriophage MS2 in 1972 [23], and the first complete 3569-nucleotide-long genome sequence of the bacteriophage MS2 RNA in 1976 [24].

Two influential techniques in the mid-1970s emerged which later gave a new dimension to the field of molecular biology. The two techniques were Alan Coulson and Sanger's "plus and minus" technique, using DNA polymerase to sequentially add radiolabeled nucleotides, and Allan Maxam and Walter Gilbert's chemical cleavage technique [25–27]. Both of these techniques moved away from 2D fractionation toward polyacrylamide gel electrophoresis, which provided better base resolution. The development of these two methods is often described as the foundation of modern sequencing but was supplanted in 1977 with Sanger's "chain termination" or "dideoxy technique," which quickly became the most widely used sequencing method over the next several decades.

The full potential of Sanger sequencing was not realized until the integration of a series of seminal improvements occurred. First, radioactive isotope labels were replaced with variably colored fluorescent tags for each nucleotide, which enabled the reaction to occur in a single vessel instead of four. A second key improvement was the use of capillary tube-based electrophoresis which provided better resolution, required less equipment space, and decreased the time required. Following these improvements, Smith et al. (1986) at Applied Biosystems Instruments™ (ABI) designed the first automated capillary sequencing system and later introduced the first commercial automated DNA sequencer [28].

These retrospectively named "first-generation" sequencers were the first to incorporate computer-based data acquisition and analysis and were capable of producing reads >300 bp. However, to analyze longer DNA molecules, "shotgun sequencing" was developed by separately cloning and sequencing overlapping DNA fragments. Coinciding with the discovery of polymerase chain reaction (PCR) and the launch of the Human Genome Project, a series of enhancements allowed machine cycle times to decrease from 18 h to 3 h [29].

In 1992, the Institute for Genomic Research (TIGR) in Rockville, Maryland, founded by J. Craig Venter, pioneered the industrialization of an automated sequencer, with a focus on studying various genomes [2, 30]. With the establishment of both the first Affymetrix® and GeneChip® microarrays in 1996, expression studies involving various genes in prokaryotes and eukaryotes were possible [31]. By the end of 1999, TIGR had generated 83 million nucleotides of cDNA sequence, 87,000 human cDNA sequences, and the complete genome sequences of *Haemophilus influenzae* [32] and *Mycoplasma genitalium* [33]. The platform resulted in the early completion of the Human Genome Project in 2003.

Next-Generation Sequencing Application

With the completion of the human genome sequence, the clinical and research appetite for comparative sequencing data expanded overnight, rapidly overwhelming the capacity and cost structure of dideoxy base sequencing. Various groups sought to bring new instruments to market (Fig. 6.1) that offered various strategies for (i) the parallelization of many sequencing reactions, (ii) the preparation of amplified sequencing libraries prior to sequencing, (iii) library amplification on miniature surfaces (solid surfaces, beads, emulsion droplets), (iv) direct monitoring of the nucleotides via advanced microfluidics and imaging, (v) reduced per-nucleotide costs, and (vi) decreased machine cycle times. However, early NGS platforms were designed to sequence entire genomes from single subjects rather than selected regions from multiple subjects. Thus, targeted sequencing for the coding regions of the genome (i.e., the exome) or regions of interest was facilitated via probe hybridization of fragmented DNA or by customized PCR amplification. Figure 6.1 highlights

Chapter 6. Advancements in Next-Generation Sequencing

common library preparation protocols, sequencing platforms, and bioinformatic considerations for performing an NGS project.

Short-read sequencing (SRS) typically produces reads that are 50–600 bp in length and has become the dominant type of NGS available today through multiple vendors (ref 34). SRS often results in scaffolding gaps due to bias from high GC content, repeat sequences, and missing insertions. There are several advantages of SRS such as high throughput, low cost

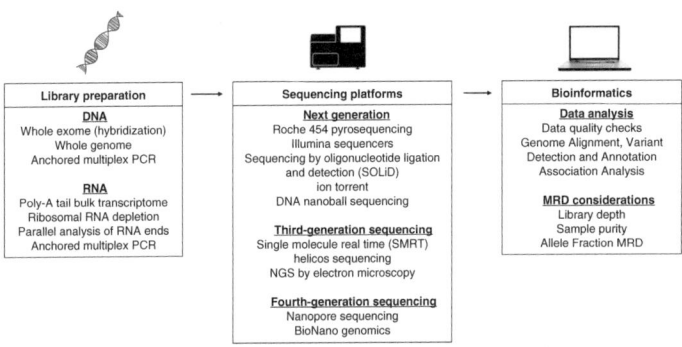

FIGURE 6.1 Overview of next-generation sequencing. *Library preparation box*: Library preparations are specific for DNA or RNA sequencing applications. Different capture techniques are available and determine what type of mutations can be captured for sequencing. *Sequencing platforms box*: The first instruments capable of performing massive parallelization of sequencing were termed next-generation sequencers. Third-generation instruments focus on long-read sequencing techniques. Fourth-generation sequencers involve unique technologies that preserve the spatial localization of the DNA/RNA molecules. *Bioinformatics box*: Raw next-generation sequencing data is unstructured and massive, requiring special analytical pipelines. When detecting minimal residual disease, it is essential to consider characteristics about the sample (purity and allele fraction MRD), sequencing technology (library depth requirements), and capture technique

per base, and a low raw read rate [35]. However, the short-read length complicates genome alignment leading to false-positive and false-negative variant calling [36, 37]. The error rate of approximately 1% primarily occurs due to dephasing of nucleotide additions (most frequently due to adding an erroneous base but can also occur due to missing base addition or adding an extra base inappropriately) to random sequences at random clusters across the flow cell, more so in the later sequencing cycles. Furthermore, de novo assembly approaches can be challenging with SRS and require enhanced algorithms for performing these operations, such as SOAPdenovo [38]. Assemble of a large genome, especially for non-model organisms, generated from SRS are limited as long-range linking information is not available [39].

In contrast, newer long-range sequencing (LRS) techniques produce reads between 10 Kb and 40 Kb [3, 4, 40, 41]. While the long read makes alignment and phasing more tractable, these platforms have historically suffered from lower total output, relatively high error rates and cost. Unfortunately, these approaches are not presently sufficient to detect very rare mutations in heterogeneous nucleic acid samples, but that may change with additional improvements.

There are several variant algorithm detection methods, including FreeBayes [42], that are specific for SRS data. The advantages for SRS for MRD include low error rate and the ability to generate deep coverage for a specific region of the genome. Therefore, SRS has dominated the field for cancer genomics as variant detection is more accurate with SRS over LRS techniques that have a higher error rate and less sensitive limit of detection. Furthermore, as error-corrected sequencing (Overview Fig. 6.2) and single-cell sequencing continue to develop, the advantages of SRS increase.

More than 70% of genetic variations seen in humans are non-SNP variations and can be missed easily with short-read sequencing [34]. Long-read sequencing enables reads longer than 10 kb, which improves alignment to the reference genome, high consensus accuracy, uniform coverage, and detection of epigenetic modifications. In addition, long-read sequencing is beneficial in transcriptomic analyses as it allows

Chapter 6. Advancements in Next-Generation Sequencing 171

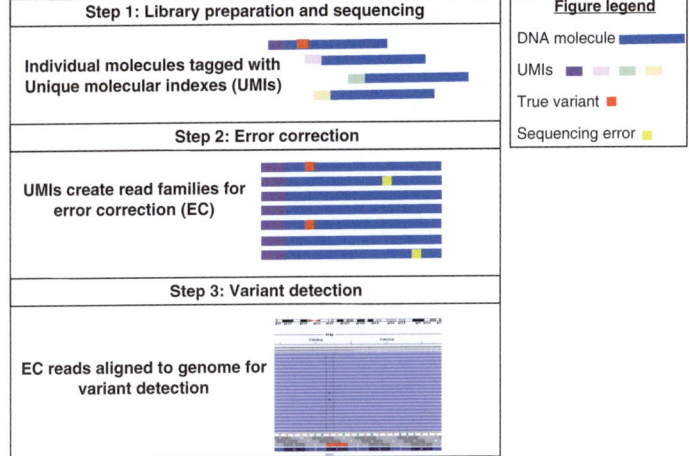

FIGURE 6.2 Workflow for error-corrected sequencing. By tagging each DNA molecule with a unique molecular index (Step 1), read families can be generated, by aligning reads with the same UMI, and used to determine sequencing errors versus low allelic variants (Step 2). Error-corrected sequences are then aligned to a reference genome and used to calculate variants (Step 3)

detection of splice isoforms with a high level of confidence without requiring assembly. High costs of long-read sequencing and high error rates are the major hurdle for adopting these platforms as a global sequencing platform.

Bioinformatics and NGS

Bioinformatics is an interdisciplinary field focused on developing methods for translating one or more large biological datasets, inherent in NGS, into applicable knowledge. Through translational computational discoveries, clinicians have gained a better understanding of genetic alterations associated with many disorders, as a priori knowledge is not required. With the publication of several best practices guidelines for NGS, basic processing steps have been well established in the scientific community (Overview Fig. 6.3).

However, as the field continues to leverage more complex NGS strategies in cancer genetics, bioinformatics has become the bottleneck in terms of expertise, infrastructure, and time to results. Currently, there is no gold standard computational pipeline that will work for all analysis, and oftentimes each project needs specific tailoring of the algorithms, which requires rigorous validation of computational processes and biological results.

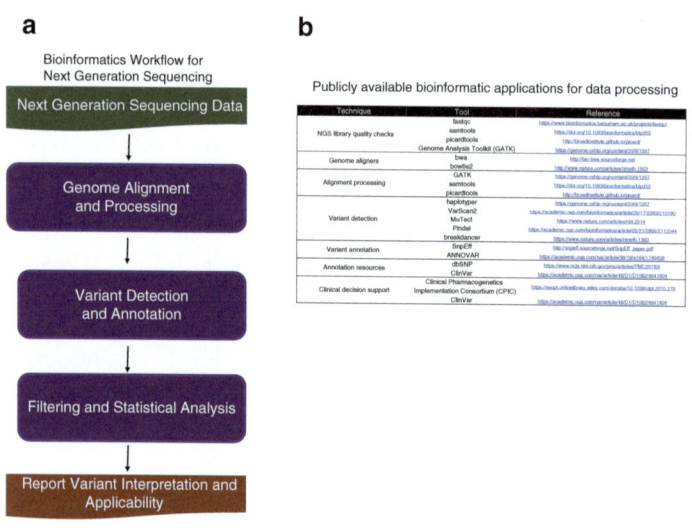

FIGURE 6.3 Bioinformatics workflow for next-generation sequencing assays. (**a**) NGS generates massive raw unstructured sequence data (green box) that is used for downstream processing. The most common file format for this data is a fastq file. The NGS reads are aligned to a reference genome and processed for variant detection annotation (purple boxes). The final output from a computational pipeline is a variant call file (VCF) that contains all of the relevant metadata per variant (dark orange box). (**b**) Numerous publicly available tools resources are available for data analysis. *maybe do a supplemental table linked here with full webpage and references? [43]

Quality Assessment of NGS Libraries

In 2012, the US Centers for Disease Control and Prevention (CDC) published the guidelines assembled by a national working group, termed Next-Generation Sequencing: Standardization of Clinical Testing or Nex-StoCT, to lead an initiative for defining platform-independent guidelines for using NGS in clinical practice [44]. The Supplementary Guidelines published by Nex-StoCT highlight key quality metrics that should be considered when establishing and validating a clinical NGS workflow. There are several publicly available tools for performing these types of quality control assessment. For example, fastqc, a platform-independent NGS quality tool (Babraham Institute, https://www.bioinformatics.babraham.ac.uk/projects/fastqc/), can import data from alignment files or raw NGS data and reports an overview of quality statistics that may indicate problems or biases in the NGS data. There are ten key statistical modules within the fastqc pipeline that report a value of "pass," "warning," or "fail" for the NGS library, consistent with the guidelines published by the CDC. We have briefly summarized each of these ten metrics below.

The sequence length, or insert size, is a basic analysis, and skewing from the expected insert size can indicate poor library construction, which needs to be carefully considered when analyzing data for novel InDels. This is a relatively simple calculation that is considered along with other basic statistics such as the total number of sequences and the maximum and minimum sequence length. The library depth is key for understanding limits of detection and should be taken into consideration during data analysis and experimental design phases. One of the remarkable aspects of genomics is its scalability. Depending upon the mutation frequency threshold (e.g., 5% vs 1% vs 0.1% or lesser) being interrogated, the sequencing strategy and library depth for an MRD assay will be quite different compared to germline sequencing requirements.

When analyzing a sample for MRD, it is essential to examine the per sequence quality scores to determine if the library has a portion of reads with low-quality values that might skew results. Ideally, poor quality reads should be a very small percentage of the total raw data. Occasionally the 3′ end of NGS reads can be of poor quality when sequencing by synthesis because sequences in a cluster can elongate at slightly different rates, which will slowly lead to desynchronizationand quality issues [45]. These low-quality bases should therefore be "trimmed" or "clipped" to help with accurate alignment and variant detection. Furthermore, overrepresented sequences are any sequences that may be overrepresented in the NGS reads, i.e., adaptors, and it is important to trim these types of sequences from the raw NGS data to improve genome alignment. Some alignment software, such as bwa-mem, enable soft clipping and can "trim" these adapter sequences during genome alignment. However, it is good practice to determine the level of adapter contamination in a library file prior to downstream analysis. Several publicly available tools, such as cutadapt [46], are established for just these purposes and improve the efficiency of downstream NGS analysis [47].

Analyzing the per base sequence content statistic is another key metric to analyze. Typically, a sample is flagged if the difference between A, T, G, or C is greater than 10% in any position. However, some targeted or enriched NGS datasets, such as exomes from hybridization capture, are known to display discreet, position-specific compositional biases [48]. In addition, nucleotide composition is known to more likely be G + C rich in first exons, and general variation basis within the genome and at the gene level are noted [49]. These known skews within coding regions can cause a targeted sequencing library to be inappropriately flagged as poor quality, so it is important to recognize the difference between targeted sequencing statistics compared to random bulk.

The per base GC content statistics calculates the GC content across the length of each sequence and compares it to a modeled normal distribution of GC content. Typically, it is important for all libraries to have the sum of the deviations from the normal distribution represented <30% of the reads.

The per base N content statistic calculates the percentage of base calls at each position for which N, or no base call, appears. A base is called "*N*" when the sequencing quality is too low to accurately call a base. The number of "*N*" bases should be limited and typically only at the 5′ or 3′ end of the reads. A library with a large portion of bases called as N indicates overall poor sequencing, and the library should be flagged and re-sequenced.

The sequence duplication level statistics counts the degree of duplication for every sequence in a library. This is important as libraries with high sequence duplication levels indicate low complexity (i.e., not sampling enough total molecules) along with a likely enrichment bias during library preparation. However, certain types of library preparations, such as RNA-seq, are known to have some bias that can lead to high duplication levels, whereas for exomes, the number of duplicated reads should be minimal. Duplicate reads can be flagged and eliminated or normalized during computational analysis to avoid false-positive variant calling and is part of the best practice guidelines for downstream processing.

The Kmer statistics measures the number of each 7-mer at each position in the library. It then uses a binomial test to look for significant deviations from an even coverage at all positions [50]. Any Kmers with a positional biased enrichment are reported. Libraries which derive from random priming can show Kmer bias at the start of the library due to an incomplete sampling of the possible random primers (Babraham Institute).

Genome Alignment and Processing

High-quality genome alignment of NGS reads is essential for accurate detection of germline, somatic, and MRD variants. There are numerous publicly available genome aligners, including but not limited to bwa-mem [51], bowtie2 [52], and FreeBayes [42], as well as de novo assembly packages that do not require forced reference mapping. Genome alignment works well for single-nucleotide variants (SNVs), small InDels, and structural variant (SV) detection when combined with pair-end data. DNA and RNA can be aligned to a genome, although RNA mapping requires an aligner capable of gapped alignment, such as tophat [53]/bowtie2 [52], due to the structure of DNA (introns) compared to RNA molecules.

The Broad Institute has developed a publicly available software package, Genome Analysis Toolkit (GATK), that provides a suite of algorithms required for processing and analyzing alignment files. GATK best practices [54] include several steps for improving genome alignment. The first step in processing the alignment files is to mark duplicate reads because they potentially represent a clonal amplification rather than a randomly sheared DNA fragment.

Next, the alignment files are analyzed for potential intervals that need realignment based on known genetic alterations. These regions undergo a realignment step for optimization. Finally, the alignment file undergoes a recalibration of base quality scores based on the adjustments from the proceeding steps. After recalibration, the quality scores, in theory, should be more accurate because the new score is closer to the actual probability of mismatching to the reference genome.

After the alignment files are appropriately processed, it is important to assess the quality of the overall genome alignment. There are several different criteria that can be used, such as percentage of reads mapped to the genome, but it is important to consider the depth and breadth of coverage. Coverage calculations are especially important when trying to understand variant calling capabilities and limitations. The depth of coverage is how many times a nucleotide was sequenced, whereas the breadth of coverage is the average coverage per base per the number of total bases queried or the sequence interval.

Variant Detection and Annotation

Single-nucleotide polymorphisms (SNPs) naturally occur between healthy individuals with estimates ranging from 1 in

1000 to 1 in 1500 nucleotides [55–57]. Collectively, SNPs result in ~3 million nucleotide differences using the estimated genome size of ~3 billion nucleotides (haploid). Additionally, somatic mutations are difficult to detect because they occur at low frequencies in the genome and might only be present in a small fraction of the DNAmolecules [58]. Often, tools used for detecting germline SNPs are not recommended for detecting SNVs. The sensitivity and specificity of an algorithm to detect a somatic mutation are dependent on several characteristics such as sequencing depth, local sequencing error rate, and allelic fraction.

There are several publicly available algorithms, including MuTect [59] and VarScan [60], for detecting somatic variants. Algorithms like MuTect simultaneously analyze both a non-cancer and cancer alignment file from the same patient, consisting of four key steps: (1) removal of low-quality sequence data, (2) variant detection in the tumor sample using a Bayesian classifier or probabilistic classifier, (3) filtering to remove false positives resulting from correlated sequencing artifacts that are not captured by the error model, and (4) designation of the variants as somatic or germline by a second Bayesian classifier.

There are multiple approaches for detecting SV using NGS data. For example, de novo assembly, with either the complete dataset or unmapped reads, is one strategy for detecting large SV [61]. One limitation to this approach is that it can only detect homozygous SV because detecting heterozygous SV requires assembly of haplotype sequences, which is a complex problem that is not fully resolved.

Reference mapping strategies are another approach and include concepts around split pair-end read mapping, read coverage depth analysis, or analysis of inconsistent insert size of paired-end reads. These approaches first require the NGS reads to be mapped to a reference genome, and then the alignment files are analyzed for genomic variants. The detection of SV using NGS data requires accurate prediction of copy, content, and structure. Often algorithms developed for detecting SVs are specific for a class of SVs, making it a necessity to incorporate multiple SV algorithms into the workflow.

Common algorithms include Pindel, BreakDancer, and VarScan2. Pindel can detect breakpoints of large deletions, medium-sized insertions, inversions, and tandem duplications by leveraging a pattern growth approach [62]. Previously, Pindel has been cited for detecting an internal tandem duplication (ITD) in the *FLT3* gene by using a pattern growth approach to analyze NGS data misaligned to the reference genome due to biological differences.

BreakDancer predicts five types of structural variants: insertions, deletions, inversions, inter- and intrachromosomal translocations, and the results from BreakDancer can be directly feed into Pindel to help enhance the analysis as a whole. VarScan2 is another package capable of detecting SVs, including copy number variations (CNVs) and InDels [63]. Ultimately, the analysis pipeline requires the integration of all of these variant callers, because leukemias are genetically heterogeneous diseases that are not characterized by a few variants or even the same class of variants.

The majority of the variant detection algorithms output a variant call file (VCF), which needs further annotation. There are several publicly available tools for performing robust somatic variant annotation, and recently the Association for Molecular Pathology published standards and guidelines for interpreting such annotations [64]. The majority of these algorithms are capable of annotating SNVs with putative functional consequences, reporting functional importance scores, and identifying previously reported SNVs and allele frequencies [64]. Oftentimes these annotations are applied in downstream filtering strategies to prioritize relevant variants. SnpEff is another publicly available algorithm for annotating VCFs [65] and provides a suite for predicting the effect of variants. Typically, researchers are interested in variants that alter the sequence of proteins, such as a missense or frameshift. However, it is noticeable that predicting whether or not a variant is damaging is still a complex issue that needs further refinement, which was recently highlighted by the Critical Assessment of Genome Interpretation (CAGI) experiments [66].

Variant Filtering and Association Analyses

NGS assays generate massive amounts of variant data, including normal population heterogeneity, sequencing artifacts, and potentially disease-associated variation. Ultimately, an effective filtering strategy for identifying disease-associated variation is required, which must be accompanied by appropriate false-negative and false-positive rates. VCF annotation packages (reviewed above) enable a researcher to build an effective filtering strategy to focus on variants that are high quality and of clinical relevance [67, 68].

Typically, filtering strategies are implemented for small sample sizes, and often more complex association statistics, like genome-wide association studies (GWAS), are not possible. Recently, several algorithms have been designed for performing associations between a set of rare variants and phenotypes from NGS data, including SNP-set (sequence) kernel association test (SKAT) [69]. Of interest, SKAT is capable of analyzing the cumulative effect of rare and common variants and is well suited for associating NGS data to a phenotype of interest.

Due to the rarity of the mutations in question, filtering strategies for MRD are complex and different compared to the filtering strategies employed to detect high-frequency somatic variants and germline variants or SNPs. Thus, while not mandatory, in order to effectively analyze MRD, it is essential to quantify the cumulative profile of low AF variants at time of diagnosis if at all possible, akin to ΔN flow cytometry, and track the presence of these and other new mutations at multiple time points post therapy.

DNA Sequencing and Applications in MRD

The three most common NGS DNA sequencing approaches in oncology are whole genome sequencing (WGS), whole exome sequencing (WES), or a targeted gene panel approach (Table 6.2). Each has strengths and weaknesses. WES enriches for sequences encoding proteins, which represents ~1–2% of the human genome [70]. WES works well for common sequence changes in coding regions, such as germline variants and high-frequency somatic mutations in cancer, but is not adequate for MRD below 2% VAF as the error rates of NGS preclude identification below that threshold (Table 6.2). More importantly, WES ignores the noncoding, regulatory regions of the genome and is incapable of detecting the breadth of mutational diversity common in cancer, such as cryptic gene fusions and complex structural variants.

WGS generates the sequence of the entire genome, not just the 1–2% in protein-coding regions. This is of obvious benefit for detecting cancer-related mutations [71]. WGS generates massive amounts of data per individual and is still fairly expensive for a clinical assay. Furthermore, the computational infrastructure required to analyze WGS is complex and beyond the majority of most clinical labs, even in the commercial space. Similar to WES, this technique works well for germline variants and detection of common somatic mutations. Beyond WES, WGS will identify duplications,

TABLE 6.2 NGS and MRD

NGS library preparation	Analyte	Advantages MRD	Disadvantage MRD	Recommended for MRD
Hybridization	DNA	Targeted assay Compatible with error correction Cheap	Limitations in variant capture for structural variants, cryptic gene fusions, and large insertions/deletions	Yes

Chapter 6. Advancements in Next-Generation Sequencing

TABLE 6.2 (continued)

NGS library preparation	Analyte	Advantages MRD	Disadvantage MRD	Recommended for MRD
Whole genome	DNA	Bulk sequencing no a priori knowledge required	Expensive Variant capture limitations Limit of detection not suited for MRD High error rate	No
Anchored multi-plex PCR (AMP)	DNA / RNA	Targeted assay Compatible with error correction Cheap Diverse variant capture	High sequencing depths required	Yes
Poly-A tail bulk transcriptome	RNA	Bulk sequencing no a priori knowledge required	High error rate Expensive for depth requirements Limitations in variant capture	No
Ribosomal RNA depletion	RNA	Bulk sequencing no a priori knowledge required	High error rate High sequencing depth required Expensive Limitations in variant capture	No
Single-cell sequencing	RNA	Robust clonal analysis	High error rate Sequencing depth requirements are cost prohibitive Limitations in variant capture	Yes

DNA fusions, inversions, large InDels, and other SVs that would not be visible by WES. However, genomes typically don't get high depth of sequencing as a cost-saving measure, which obviates their utility for MRD (Table 6.2). For both WES and WGS, two critical considerations in the clinical space are whether they are reimbursed by third-party payors and what is the obligation of the individual ordering the test to relate incidental findings. For these reasons, many third-party payors refuse payment, and many clinicians are reticent to order tests that are much more broad in scope than the cancer-related question at hand. However, some academic centers have established genetic counseling services or other protocols to relate the transfer of incidental genetic findings to patients and families.

For MRD, targeted panels are currently better suited due to being more customizable for specific disease-related loci and cost-efficacy. Targeted panels use a variety of strategies to enrich for target sequences such as nucleic acid hybridization, rolling circle amplification, molecular inversion probes, and various PCR-based enrichment strategies. Each has advantages and disadvantages, but the main metric is "on/off target" percentage. At the best of times, these various strategies (other than plain PCR) only "capture" somewhere between 2 and 7% of the molecules available. For MRD, this needs to be taken into careful consideration. For example, to detect a mutation at 0.0001 (1:10,000), one needs to query at least 10,000 different molecules. If one starts with 5,000,000 molecules (~8.2 μg) and 95% are not captured, that leaves 250,000 molecules, so a mutation at 0.0001 should be seen 25 times. Obviously, the amount of starting material becomes substantial, and often rate-limiting, quite quickly.

Error-Corrected DNA Sequencing

Given that leukemias are a heterogenous mixture of subclones [72], error-corrected sequencing (ECS) enables the tagging of a single DNA molecule with a unique molecular index [72–75]. Utilizing this approach, stochastic errors are introduced by the sequencing platforms. As demonstrated by Young et al. [73], targeted gene panels incorporating a unique molecular index are capable of detecting clonal hematopoiesis involving known oncogenes in healthy adults [73].

The main aspects of error-corrected sequencing as described by Young et al. are (i) aggregating all of the reads arising from a single molecule as demonstrated by sharing the same random index (e.g., "read family") to computationally subtract stochastic sequencing artifacts and (ii) an analysis of the error rate at each base by establishing a negative binomial distribution. Read family aggregation into a single "error-corrected consensus sequence" is done prior to genome alignment. After variant detection, a second analysis can be done to calculate the error rate at each position and further filter variants to remove false positives that are actually sequencing artifacts [73].

Different ECS strategies must be implemented to identify SNVs and/or InDels at low allelic frequencies [73, 76] compared to SVs. Precise quantification of SVs in DNA involves amplifying a target locus with many different amplification primers on each side of the putative lesion or breakpoint. This results in many possible amplicons, which can then be aligned via de novo assembly rather than forced reference alignment. A major aspect of applying this technology for MRD (Table 6.2) is the ability to link the data to either an earlier time point from the same subject, and to connect the variants of interest to external resources for rigors filtering strategies.

RNA Sequencing and Applications in MRD

Various library techniques exist for RNA sequencing, including poly-A tail capture for mRNA, ribosomal RNA depletion, parallel analysis of RNA ends (PARE-seq), and targeted gene panels [77, 78]. Bulk RNA sequencing techniques process thousands of cells at once and represent the "average" of all of the molecules within the mixed population sequenced.

The traditional analysis for RNA-seq was differential gene expression, but over the last several years, the community has developed extensive computational pipelines for detecting variants [79].

RNA sequencing enables the detection of several variant classes that are not easily detectable via DNA sequencing, including cryptic gene fusions, exon usage, and allele-specific expression. These types of variants are quickly being associated with various cancers [80] and are of interest for MRD applications [81] either alone or in combination with other diagnostic tools. Poddighe et al. (2018) recently developed an MRD assay for CBFB-MYH11 gene fusion. Interestingly, the fusion was also detected at time of birth in the same subject when analyzing cord blood [81] highlighting the growing realization that "cancer-related" mutations are far more common in the general population than previously appreciated (Young AL et al., *Nat Commun* 2016) because only ill people have historically undergone such careful analyses. As capture techniques and computational pipelines continue to improve our ability to detect these types of variants, our understanding of their biology is quickly changing.

Similar to gene panels for DNA sequencing, targeted RNA gene panel sequencing strategies enable an in-depth analysis of transcripts of interest. A PCR amplification strategy, single or opposing primers, enables the capture of cryptic gene fusions and will hopefully help to improve our understanding of intron retention in cancer patients [82]. Targeted RNA panels also have the advantage, compared to bulk sequencing methods, of incorporating unique molecular indexes, which enables error correction.

Error-Corrected RNA Sequencing

Similar to DNA-ECS, RNA-ECS is currently best applied to targeted gene panels. In contrast, the RNA-ECS consensus read family sequence is aligned to the genome using a gap reference aligner and analyzed for small InDels and SNVs.

For more complex variants, including cryptic gene fusions, alternative exon usage, structural variants, and novel transcript structure, such as retained intron, a de novo assembly approach from multiple, variably sized amplicons across the breakpoint is required [83], compared to a force reference alignment. There are several publicly available de novo assemblers available for this type of work, such as ABySS [84]. One major limitation of ECS, whether for RNA or DNA, is the inability to co-localize mutations within the same cellular background. The identified clonal mutations are often so rare that (a) the overall difference in the abundance and genes that are mutated between heathy and diseased individuals is minimal, (b) making the likelihood of multiple mutations co-occurring to be statistically highly unlikely, but biologically critical. One could imagine new mutations being identified serially in a patient treated for leukemia. The effect size of these new mutations may range from negligible, if occurring alone at a low frequency, to catastrophic, if co-occurring in a clone or subclone of the original leukemia. ECS can only make inferences as to the relatively likelihood of mutational co-occurrence.

Single-Cell Sequencing

Against this context, the field of cancer genomics will quickly transition to sequencing techniques that enable the genomic or epigenomic characterization of an individual cell, providing higher resolution of co-occurring mutations within the same cell and have even lead to the discovery of new cell types [85]. Processing for single-cell RNA sequencing (sc-RNA-seq) is quite different than traditional transcriptome sequencing. Currently, RNA preservation is key such that the first step is isolation of viable, single cells from the tissue of interest. For dissociation of single cells from solid tumors, this can effect RNA quality and requires special handling procedures compared to storage for DNA sequencing projects.

The application of sc-RNA-seq for MRD has not yet been fully realized because current RNA sequencing on these platforms only queries dozens of bases at the 3′ end of an mRNA molecule. Thus, it is quite good at quantifying transcripts but cannot uniformly quantify mutations residing further upstream in the mRNA molecule. As these technologies mature and become more amenable to MRD analyses, it will be important to consider sequencing depth requirements and number of cells assayed [86].

References

1. BBC NEWS | science/nature | what they said: genome in quotes.
2. Kulski JK. Next-generation sequencing — an overview of the history, tools, and "Omic" applications; 2016
3. Levy SE, Myers RM. Advancements in next-generation sequencing. Annu Rev Genomics Hum Genet. 2016;17(1):95–115.
4. Srinivasan S, Batra J. Four generations of sequencing- is it ready for the clinic yet? J Next Gener Seq Appl. 2014;1:107.
5. Ari Ş, Arikan M. Next-generation sequencing: advantages, disadvantages, and future. In: Plant omics: trends and applications. Cham: Springer; 2016. p. 109–35.
6. Nowell PC. The clonal evolution of tumor cell populations. Science. 1976;194(4260):23–8.
7. Fan J, Han F, Liu H. Challenges of big data analysis. Natl Sci Rev. 2014;1(2):293–314.
8. Kruglyak KM, Lin E, Ong FS. Next-generation sequencing and applications to the diagnosis and treatment of lung Cancer. Adv Exp Med Biol. 2016;890:123–36.
9. https://dx.doi.org/10.1093%2Fnar%2Fgks1443.
10. Walter FM, Emery JD. Genetic advances in medicine: has the promise been fulfilled in general practice? Br J Gen Pract. 2012;62(596):120–1.
11. Landau DA, Carter SL, Getz G, Wu CJ. Clonal evolution in hematological malignancies and therapeutic implications. Leukemia. 2014;28(1):34.
12. Niederhuber J, Armitage J, Doroshow J, Kastan M, Tepper J. Abeloff's clinical oncology. 5th ed. Philadelphia: Saunders; 2013. p. 2224.

13. The molecular landscape of pediatric acute myeloid leukemia reveals recurrent structural alterations and age-specific mutational interactions | nature medicine.
14. THE CHROMOSOME NUMBER OF MAN - TJIO - 1956 - Hereditas - Wiley Online Library.
15. Speicher MR, Carter NP. The new cytogenetics: blurring the boundaries with molecular biology. Nat Rev Genet. 2005;6(10):782.
16. Pui C-H, Carroll WL, Meshinchi S, Arceci RJ. Biology, risk stratification, and therapy of pediatric acute Leukemias: an update. J Clin Oncol. 2011;29(5):551–65.
17. Admin. The history of DNA timeline. DNA worldwide. 2014.
18. Holley RW, Apgar J, Everett GA, Madison JT, Marquisee M, Merrill SH, et al. Structure of a ribonucleic acid. Science (80-). 1965;147(3664):1462–5.
19. Buermans HPJ, den Dunnen JT. Next generation sequencing technology: advances and applications. Biochim Biophys Acta Mol basis Dis. 2014;1842(10):1932–41.
20. Heather JM, Chain B. The sequence of sequencers: the history of sequencing DNA. Genomics. 2016;107(1):1–8.
21. Sanger F, Brownlee GG. Barrell BG. A two-dimensional fractionation procedure for radioactive nucleotides. J Mol Biol. 1965;13(2):373–98.
22. Wu R, Kaiser AD. Structure and base sequence in the cohesive ends of bacteriophage lambda DNA. J Mol Biol. 1968;35(3):523–37.
23. Jou WM, Haegeman G, Ysebaert M, Fiers W. Nucleotide sequence of the gene coding for the bacteriophage MS2 coat protein. Nature. 1972;237(5350):82.
24. Fiers W, Contreras R, Duerinck F, Haegeman G, Iserentant D, Merregaert J, et al. Complete nucleotide sequence of bacteriophage MS2 RNA: primary and secondary structure of the replicase gene. Nature. 1976;260(5551):500.
25. Sanger F, Coulson AR. A rapid method for determining sequences in DNA by primed synthesis with DNA polymerase. J Mol Biol. 1975;94(3):441–8.
26. Sanger F, Air GM, Barrell BG, Brown NL, Coulson AR, Fiddes JC, et al. Nucleotide sequence of bacteriophage φX174 DNA. Nature. 1977;265(5596):687.
27. Maxam AM, Gilbert W. A new method for sequencing DNA. Proc Natl Acad Sci U S A. 1977;74(2):560–4.

28. Smith LM, Sanders JZ, Kaiser RJ, Hughes P, Dodd C, Connell CR, et al. Fluorescence detection in automated DNA sequence analysis. Nature. 1986;321(6071):674.
29. Ansorge WJ. Next-generation DNA sequencing techniques. New Biotechnol. 2009;25(4):195–203.
30. Adams MD, Kelley JM, Gocayne JD, Dubnick M, Polymeropoulos MH, Xiao H, et al. Complementary DNA sequencing: expressed sequence tags and human genome project. Science (80-). 1991;252(5013):1651–6.
31. Bumgarner R. Overview of DNA microarrays: types, applications, and their future. Curr Protoc Mol Biol. 2013; Chapter 22:Unit 22.1. doi: https://doi.org/10.1002/0471142727.mb2201s101.
32. Fleischmann RD, Adams MD, White O, Clayton RA, Kirkness EF, Kerlavage AR, et al. Whole-genome random sequencing and assembly of Haemophilus influenzae Rd. Science (80-). 1995;269(5223):496–512.
33. Fraser CM, Gocayne JD, White O, Adams MD, Clayton RA, Fleischmann RD, et al. The minimal gene complement of mycoplasma genitalium. Science (80-). 1995;270(5235):397–404.
34. A map of human genome variation from population scale sequencing. Nature. 2010;467(7319):1061–73.
35. Caspar SM, Dubacher N, Kopps AM, Meienberg J, Henggeler C, Matyas G. Clinical sequencing: from raw data to diagnosis with lifetime value. Clin Genet:n/a–a.
36. Derrien T, Estellé J, Sola SM, Knowles DG, Raineri E, Guigó R, et al. Fast computation and applications of genome Mappability. PLoS One. 2012;7(1):e30377.
37. Mandelker D, Schmidt RJ, Ankala A, Gibson KM, Bowser M, Sharma H, et al. Navigating highly homologous genes in a molecular diagnostic setting: a resource for clinical next-generation sequencing. Genet Med. 2016;18(12):1282.
38. Li R, Zhu H, Ruan J, Qian W, Fang X, Shi Z, et al. De novo assembly of human genomes with massively parallel short read sequencing. Genome Res. 2010;20(2):265–72.
39. The Long and the Short of DNA Sequencing. GEN.
40. Liu L, Li Y, Li S, Hu N, He Y, Pong R, et al. Comparison of next-generation sequencing systems. Bio Med Res Int. 2012;2012:251364.
41. Illumina | sequencing and array-based solutions for genetic research.
42. Garrison E. Freebayes: Bayesian haplotype-based genetic polymorphism discovery and genotyping; 2018.

43. Wang K, Li M, Hakonarson H. ANNOVAR: Functional annotation of genetic variants from high-throughput sequencing data. Nucleic Acids Res. 2010;38(16):e164.
44. Gargis AS, Kalman L, Berry MW, Bick DP, Dimmock DP, Hambuch T, et al. Assuring the quality of next-generation sequencing in clinical laboratory practice. Nat Biotechnol [Internet]. 2012;30(11):1033–6. Available from: http://www.nature.com/articles/nbt.2403.
45. https://doi.org/10.1038/nbt.1585.
46. Martin M. Cutadapt removes adapter sequences from high-throughput sequencing reads. EMBnet J. 2011;17(1):10–2.
47. Del FC, Scalabrin S, Morgante M, Giorgi FM. An extensive evaluation of read trimming effects on Illumina NGS data analysis. PLoS One. 2013;8(12):e85024.
48. Kozlowski P, de Mezer M, Krzyzosiak WJ. Trinucleotide repeats in human genome and exome. Nucleic Acids Res [Internet]. 2010;38(12):4027–39. Available from: https://academic.oup.com/nar/article-lookup/doi/10.1093/nar/gkq127.
49. Louie E, Ott J, Majewski J. Nucleotide frequency variation across human genes. Genome Res. 2003;13(12):2594–601.
50. Babraham Institute, https://www.bioinformatics.babraham.ac.uk/projects/fastqc/.
51. Burrows-Wheeler Aligner.
52. Bowtie 2: fast and sensitive read alignment.
53. Trapnell C, Pachter L, Salzberg SL. TopHat: discovering splice junctions with RNA-Seq. Bioinformatics. 2009;25(9):1105–11.
54. DePristo MA, Banks E, Poplin R, Garimella KV, Maguire JR, Hartl C, et al. A framework for variation discovery and genotyping using next-generation DNA sequencing data. Nat Genet [Internet]. 2011;43(5):491–8. Available from: http://www.nature.com/articles/ng.806.
55. Schneider JA, Pungliya MS, Choi JY, Jiang R, Sun XJ, Salisbury BA, et al. DNA variability of human genes. Mech Ageing Dev [Internet]. 2003;124(1):17–25. Available from: http://www.ncbi.nlm.nih.gov/pubmed/12618002.
56. Sachidanandam R, Weissman D, Schmidt SC, Kakol JM, Stein LD, Marth G, et al. A map of human genome sequence variation containing 1.42 million single nucleotide polymorphisms. Nature [Internet]. 2001;409(6822):928–33. Available from: http://www.nature.com/doifinder/10.1038/35057149.

57. Jorde LB, Wooding SP. Genetic variation, classification and "race". Nat Genet [Internet]. 2004;36(11s):S28–33. Available from: http://www.nature.com/doifinder/10.1038/ng1435.
58. Cibulskis K, Lawrence MS, Carter SL, Sivachenko A, Jaffe D, Sougnez C, et al. Sensitive detection of somatic point mutations in impure and heterogeneous cancer samples. Nat Biotechnol [Internet]. 2013;31(3):213–9. Available from: http://www.nature.com/doifinder/10.1038/nbt.2514.
59. Cibulskis K, Lawrence MS, Carter SL, Sivachenko A, Jaffe D, Sougnez C, et al. Sensitive detection of somatic point mutations in impure and heterogeneous cancer samples. Nat Biotechnol. 2013;31(3):213.
60. Koboldt DC, Zhang Q, Larson DE, Shen D, McLellan MD, Lin L, et al. VarScan 2: somatic mutation and copy number alteration discovery in cancer by exome sequencing. Genome Res. 2012;22(3):568–76.
61. Li Y, Zhang Q, Yin X, Yang W, Du Y, Hou P, et al. Generation of iPSCs from mouse fibroblasts with a single gene, Oct4 and small molecules. Cell Res [Internet]. 2011;21(1):196–204. Available from: http://www.nature.com/articles/cr2010142.
62. Ye K, Schulz MH, Long Q, Apweiler R, Ning Z. Pindel: a pattern growth approach to detect break points of large deletions and medium sized insertions from paired-end short reads. Bioinformatics [Internet]. 2009;25(21):2865–71. Available from: https://academic.oup.com/bioinformatics/article-lookup/doi/10.1093/bioinformatics/btp394.
63. Koboldt DC, Zhang Q, Larson DE, Shen D, McLellan MD, Lin L, et al. VarScan 2: Somatic mutation and copy number alteration discovery in Cancer by exome sequencing. Genome Res [Internet]. 2012;22(3):568–76. Available from: http://genome.cshlp.org/cgi/doi/10.1101/gr.129684.111.
64. https://doi.org/10.1016/j.jmoldx.2016.10.002.
65. Cingolani P, Platts A, Wang LL, Coon M, Nguyen T, Wang L, et al. A program for annotating and predicting the effects of single nucleotide polymorphisms, SnpEff. Fly (Austin) [Internet]. 2012;6(2):80–92. Available from: http://www.tandfonline.com/doi/abs/10.4161/fly.19695.
66. https://doi.org/10.1002/humu.23290.
67. Carson AR, Smith EN, Matsui H, Brækkan SK, Jepsen K, Hansen J-B, et al. Effective filtering strategies to improve data quality from population-based whole exome sequencing studies. BMC Bioinf. 2014;15:125.

68. Yost SE, Smith EN, Schwab RB, Bao L, Jung H, Wang X, et al. Identification of high-confidence somatic mutations in whole genome sequence of formalin-fixed breast cancer specimens. Nucleic Acids Res. 2012;40(14):e107.
69. Ionita-Laza I, Lee S, Makarov V, Buxbaum JD, Lin X. Sequence kernel association tests for the combined effect of rare and common variants. Am J Hum Genet. 2013;92(6):841–53.
70. Wang Z, Liu X, Yang B-Z, Gelernter J. The role and challenges of exome sequencing in studies of human diseases. Front Genet. 2013;4:160.
71. Sharma S, Kelly TK, Jones PA. Epigenetics in cancer. Carcinogenesis. 2010;31(1):27–36.
72. Schmitt MW, Fox EJ, Prindle MJ, Reid-Bayliss KS, True LD, Radich JP, et al. Sequencing small genomic targets with high efficiency and extreme accuracy. Nat Methods. 2015;12(5):423.
73. Young AL, Challen GA, Birmann BM, Druley TE. Clonal haematopoiesis harbouring AML-associated mutations is ubiquitous in healthy adults. Nat Commun. 2016;7:12484.
74. Kinde I, Wu J, Papadopoulos N, Kinzler KW, Vogelstein B. Detection and quantification of rare mutations with massively parallel sequencing. Proc Natl Acad Sci. 2011;108(23):9530–5.
75. Schmitt MW, Kennedy SR, Salk JJ, Fox EJ, Hiatt JB, Loeb LA. Detection of ultra-rare mutations by next-generation sequencing. Proc Natl Acad Sci. 2012;109(36):14508–13.
76. Zheng Z, Liebers M, Zhelyazkova B, Cao Y, Panditi D, Lynch KD, Chen J, Robinson HE, Shim HS, Chmielecki J, Pao W, Engelman JA, Iafrate AJ, Le LP. Anchored multiplex PCR for targeted next-generation sequencing. Nat Med. 2014;20(12):1479–84. https://doi.org/10.1038/nm.3729.
77. German MA, Pillay M, Jeong D-H, Hetawal A, Luo S, Janardhanan P, et al. Global identification of microRNA–target RNA pairs by parallel analysis of RNA ends. Nat Biotechnol. 2008;26(8):941.
78. Zhao W, He X, Hoadley KA, Parker JS, Hayes DN, Perou CM. Comparison of RNA-Seq by poly (a) capture, ribosomal RNA depletion, and DNA microarray for expression profiling. BMC Genomics. 2014;15:419.
79. Piskol R, Ramaswami G, Li JB. Reliable identification of genomic variants from RNA-Seq data. Am J Hum Genet. 2013;93(4):641–51.
80. https://www.medscape.com/viewarticle/555206.

81. Poddighe PJ, Veening MA, Mansur MB, Loonen AH, Westers TM, Merle PA, et al. A novel cryptic CBFB-MYH11 gene fusion present at birth leading to acute myeloid leukemia and allowing molecular monitoring for minimal residual disease. Hum Pathol Case Reports. 2018;11(Supplement C):34–8.
82. Dvinge H, Bradley RK. Widespread intron retention diversifies most cancer transcriptomes. Genome Med. 2015;7:45.
83. Robertson G, Schein J, Chiu R, Corbett R, Field M, Jackman SD, et al. *De novo* assembly and analysis of RNA-seq data. Nat Methods. 2010;7(11):909.
84. Birol I, Jackman SD, Nielsen CB, Qian JQ, Varhol R, Stazyk G, et al. De novo transcriptome assembly with ABySS. Bioinformatics. 2009;25(21):2872–7.
85. Villani A-C, Satija R, Reynolds G, Sarkizova S, Shekhar K, Fletcher J, et al. Single-cell RNA-seq reveals new types of human blood dendritic cell, monocytes, and progenitors. Science (80-). 2017;356(6335):eaah4573.
86. Haque A, Engel J, Teichmann SA, Lönnberg T. A practical guide to single-cell RNA-sequencing for biomedical research and clinical applications. Genome Med. 2017;9:75.

Index

A
Acute lymphoblastic leukemia
  (ALL), 23
  adverse prognostic effect, 53
  chemotherapeutic treatment
    regimens, 24
  clinical studies, PCR and flow
    cytometry, 40, 41
  flow cytometry, 30, 33
    advantages and
      disadvantages, 39, 40
    panels, 35, 36
  MRD, 25–27, 29
    surrogate marker, 55
  MRD detection, risk
    stratification and the
    threshold for, 44–53
  NGS, 41
  PCR, 36, 37
    advantages and
      disadvantages, 37, 39
  phenotypic switch and
    drug-induced
    immunophenotypic
    modulation, 34, 35
  prognostic markers for, 24
  redefine response, using
    MRD, 54, 55
  risk factors, 24
Acute myeloid leukemia
  (AML), 102
  "difference from normal"
    (ΔN), 101, 103
  flow cytometry
    assay validation, 115, 118,
      119
    correlative validation,
      123, 124
    definition of normal, 103,
      104, 106–109
    ΔN post-HSCT, direct
      validation of, 119–122
    indirect validation,
      125–127, 129, 130
    lower level of detection,
      112, 114, 116
    mutations affect
      phenotypic expression,
      110, 111
    performance
      characteristics, 113, 114,
      117
    risk stratification,
      131, 132
    specimen composition and
      quality, 111, 112
  hematopoietic malignancies,
    90, 91
  monoclonal antibody, 105
Acute promyelocytic leukemia
  (APL), 74
Affymetrix®, 5, 168

AML, *see* Acute myeloid
    leukemia
Antibodies, 38
Applied Biosystems
    Instruments™
    (ABI), 9, 167

B

B-cell acute lymphoblastic
    leukemia (B-ALL),
    24–26, 30, 34, 35, 40, 54
  NGS in, 42, 43
B-cell malignancies, 91, 92
B-cell maturation pattern, 33
BCL1 RQ-PCR, 80
BCL2 RQ-PCR, 80
BCR-ABL1, 70, 73, 74
Bioinformatics, NGS, 170, 171
  genome alignment and
      processing, 175, 176
  quality assessment of, 173–175
  variant detection and
      annotation, 177, 178
  variant filtering and
      association analyses, 179
BioNano's next-generation
    mapping, 15

C

Cancer genomics, 7, 160, 170, 183
Capillary electrophoresis
    sequencer, 83
CD34, 107, 113
CD45, 104, 106, 108, 109
CD56, 148
Chain-termination technique,
    4, 167
Chemical cleavage technique,
    3, 167
Chromatography, 3, 166
Clinical trials, 56, 78, 125, 131,
    142, 144
Core-binding factor (CBF)
    transcription factor, 76

Core-binding factor AML
    (CBF-AML), 75, 76
Correlative assay validation, 118
Correlative validation, 123, 124
Cytogenetics, 1, 24, 70, 123, 131,
    140, 165

D

Deep molecular remission
    testing, 74
Dexamethasone, cytarabine,
    6-thioguanine,
    etoposide, and
    rubidomycin/
    daunomycin
    (DCTER), 142
Dideoxy technique, 4, 167
Dideoxynucleotides (ddNTPs), 4
"Difference from normal" (ΔN),
    99
Direct assay validation, 116, 118
Direct validation of, 119–122
DNA nanoball sequencing
    (DNBS), 10, 11
DNA sequencing, 2–6, 180, 182
  ECS, 182
  history of, 166
Down syndrome (DS), 133, 145,
    148
Drug-induced
    immunophenotypic
    modulation, 33–35

E

Electron microscopy, next-
    generation sequencing,
    12, 13
Electron Optica, 13
Electrophoresis, 3, 4, 83, 86, 167
Error-corrected sequencing
    (ECS), 171
  DNA sequencing, 182, 183
  ML-DS, 150–153
  RNA sequencing, 184, 185

F

FACS immunoglobulin (Ig), 82–84, 86
First-generation sequencers, 4, 167
Flow cytometric cell sorting (FACS), 77, 81, 82
Flow cytometry, 1, 30, 33, 43, 101
  advantages and disadvantages, 39
  AML
    assay validation, 115, 118, 119
    correlative validation, 123, 124
    definition of normal, 103, 104, 106–109
    ΔN post-HSCT, direct validation of, 119–122
    indirect validation, 125–127, 129, 130
    lower level of detection, 112, 114, 116
    mutations affect phenotypic expression, 110, 111
    performance characteristics, 113, 114, 117
    risk stratification, 131, 132
    specimen composition and quality, 111, 112
  antibodies used in, 38
  clinical studies, 40, 41
Flow cytometry panels, 35, 36
Fluorescence-activated cell sorting (FACS), 148
Fluorescence in situ hybridization (FACS-FISH), 86, 87, 89
Fourth-generation sequencing, 13
FreeBayes, 7, 170, 175
French-American-British (FAB) classification, 161

G

GATA1, 140, 151, 152
GC content, 7, 169, 174
Genetic instability, 160, 165
Genome Analysis Toolkit (GATK), 176
454 GS FLX titanium system, 8

H

Helicos sequencing system, 12
Hematopoietic malignancies
  AML, 90, 91
  B-and T-cell malignancies, 91, 92
  BCL1 and BCL2 RQ-PCR, 80
  BCR-ABL1, 70, 73, 74
  CBF-AML, 75, 76
  emerging and patient-specific technique, 81
  FACS, 81, 82
  FACS Ig and TCR gene rearrangements, 82, 84
  FACS-FISH, 86, 87, 89
  Inv(16), 77, 78
  MLL, 78, 79
  molecular analysis, 92
  NGS, 90
  PML-RARA, 74, 75
  RQ-PCR, 70, 71
  t(8;21)(q22;q22.1), 76, 77
  WT1 expression, 79
High-throughput sequencing (HTS), 43, 91, 92
Human Genome Project, 163, 164, 168

I

Illumina (Solexa) sequencers, 7, 9
Immunofluorescence, 111, 124
Immunophenotypes, 144, 146, 148
Indirect assay validation, 119
Indirect validation, 125–127, 129
Internal tandem duplication (ITD), 178

Inv(16), 76–78, 140
Ion Torrent technology, 10

L

Leukemia-associated immunophenotype (LAIP) technique, 33–34, 86–87, 102
Leukemic B lymphoblasts, 36
Long-read sequencing (LRS) techniques, 7, 170
Low-energy electron microscopy (LEEM), 13

M

Megakaryoblast cells, 140
Minimal residual disease (MRD), 1, 17
    ALL, 25–27, 29
    methods, 29, 31–32
Multidimensional flow cytometry (MDF), ML-DS, 143–146, 148
Multiparameter flow cytometry (MFC), 69, 76
MuTect, 177
Myeloid leukemia of Down syndrome (ML-DS), 139
    error-corrected NGS, 150–153
    genotypic analysis, 149
    MDF, 143–146, 148
    minimizing treatment-related toxicity, 142, 143
    MRD monitoring, 141
    natural history, 140
Mylotarg®, 125

N

Nanopore sequencing, 14–15
Next-generation sequencing (NGS), 6–8, 150, 159, 169
    ALL, 41
    application, 168, 170
    in B-ALL, 42, 43
    bioinformatics and, 171
        genome alignment and processing, 175, 176
        NGS libraries, quality assessment of, 173–175
        variant detection and annotation, 177, 178
        variant filtering and association analyses, 179
    by electron microscopy, 12, 13
    hematopoietic malignancies, 90
    ML-DS, 150–153
    and MRD, 180–181
    Standardization of Clinical Testing (Nex-StoCT), 173
    in T-ALL, 41
Non-DS AML, post-induction chemotherapy regeneration, 147
Non-Hodgkin's lymphoma (NHL), 80, 92

O

Oxford Nanopore Technologies (ONT), 14, 15

P

PacBio machines, 12
Personal Genome Machine (PGM), 10
Phenotypic switch, 33–35
Plus and minus technique, 3, 167
PML-RARA, 74, 75
Polyacrylamide gel electrophoresis, 3
Polymerase chain reaction (PCR), 5, 36, 37, 168
    clinical studies, 40, 41

R

Real-time quantitative RT-PCR (RQ-PCR), 70, 71
  BCL1, 80
  BCL2, 80
RNA sequencing, 183, 184
  ECS, 184, 185
Roche 454 pyrosequencing, 8, 9
RUNX1-RUNX1T1 fusion transcripts, 76

S

Sequencing history, 161–165
Sequencing by ligation (SBL) strategy, 9
Short-read sequencing (SRS) technologies, 7, 169
Short tandem repeat analysis (STR), 118
Single-cell sequencing (SCS), 16, 17, 185, 186
Single-molecule real-time (SMRT) technology, 11
Single-nucleotide polymorphisms (SNPs), 176–177
SNP-set (sequence) kernel association test (SKAT), 179
Solid-state nanopore, 14
Supported oligonucleotide ligation and detection (SOLiD), 9–10

T

t(8;21)(q22;q22.1), 76, 77
Targeted panels, 6, 182
T-cell malignancies, 91, 92
T-cell receptor (TCR) gene rearrangements, 82–84, 86
Third-generation sequencing, 11, 163
T-lymphoblastic leukemia (T-ALL), 24–26, 30, 37, 41
  NGS in, 41
Transcriptomics, 170
Transient abnormal myelopoiesis (TAM), 140
Transient myeloproliferative disease (TMD), 139, 140, 151, 152
Transmembrane protein channels, 14
Trisomy 21, 151, 152
Tumorigenesis, 160, 165

V

Variant call file (VCF), 172, 178

W

Whole exome sequencing (WES), 180
Whole genome sequencing (WGS), 180
WT1 expression, 79

Z

Zero-mode waveguides (ZMWs), 11
ZS Genetics, 13

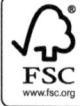

MIX
Papier aus verantwortungsvollen Quellen
Paper from responsible sources
FSC® C105338

If you have any concerns about our products,
you can contact us on
ProductSafety@springernature.com

In case Publisher is established outside the EU,
the EU authorized representative is:
**Springer Nature Customer Service Center GmbH
Europaplatz 3, 69115 Heidelberg, Germany**

Printed by Libri Plureos GmbH
in Hamburg, Germany